G. Bayer, F. Kistler, S. Kistler, S. Adler, J. Neugebauer

Immediate restorations with a reduced number of implants
Conceptual background and clinical results

G. Bayer, F. Kistler, S. Kistler, S. Adler, J. Neugebauer

Immediate restorations with a reduced number of implants

Conceptual background and clinical results

With the collaboration of:
Fabian Sigmund, Landsberg, Germany
Dr Ing. Freimut Vizethum, Rauenberg, Germany
Dr Michael Weiss, Ulm, Germany

With a foreword by:
Dr Phil Bennett

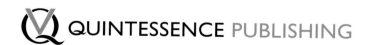

London, Berlin, Chicago, Tokyo, Barcelona, Beijing, Istanbul, Milan, Moscow, New Delhi, Paris, Prague, São Paulo, Seoul, Singapore and Warsaw

Translated from the original in German titled *Sofortversorgung mit reduzierter Implantatanzahl: Wissenschaftliche Konzeption und klinische Ergebnisse* (ISBN: 978-3-86867-048-6).

British Library Cataloguing in Publication Data

Immediate restorations with a reduced number of implants:
   conceptual background and clinical results.
   1. Maxillofacial prosthesis. 2. Dental implants.
   I. Bayer, G.
   617.5'22-dc22

ISBN: 978-1-85097-217-4

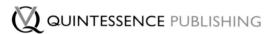

Quintessence Publishing Co., Ltd,
Grafton Road, New Malden,
Surrey KT3 3AB, Great Britain
www.quintpub.co.uk

Reproductions: DUOTONE Medienproduktion, Munich
Production: Quintessenz Verlags-GmbH, Berlin
Editorial office: Quintessenz Verlags-GmbH, Berlin
Printing: Bosch Druck GmbH, Landshut/Ergolding
Printed in Germany

Foreword

The authors of this book are well known in Germany and indeed throughout Europe. I have had the privilege of working with Dr Georg Bayer on more than one occasion, so a text written for such a specific subject must be of importance and interest to any forward-thinking implant dentist.

Populations in the developed world are getting older: this trend has characterized the aging demographic for over 100 years in the UK and most of the developed world. Population aging is defined as the process by which older individuals, that is, people aged 50 or over, make up a proportionally larger share of the total population over a period of time.

In the UK in 1901, nearly one person in seven (approximately 15%) was aged 50 and over. This increased to one in three by 2003 and is still rising. By 2031 it is projected that over 40% of the total population will be aged 50 and over[1].

The implication of the aging population is the ever increasing requirement for reconstructive dentistry in the partially or fully edentulous patient. The requirement for better quality dentistry is driven by the population of "baby boomers", whose expectations are higher than those of their forbears. Indeed, the provision of acrylic full dentures is almost an anathema to some. The production of this book will guide the way to achieving the fixed restorations that an increasing number of patients will demand.

Traditionally, the ability to reconstruct seriously damaged hard and soft tissue required multiple interventions, and a high degree of experience from the operators and a great deal of time. The authors have managed to link together the modern techniques of treatment planning using CT/DVT imaging, a well-tried implant system in the blueSKY system, a surgical approach well documented by people such as Paulo Maló and, above all, the SKY fast & fixed system, which allows for an immediate fixed solution as desired by the aging population. It is also important to point out that this treatment can be achieved for the patient at a greatly reduced cost compared with traditional reconstructions due to considerably reduced chair time and healing intervals.

The text is written in almost a step-by-step way, which will help the less experienced implant dentist, beautifully illustrated with numerous color photographs, and includes a host of practical tips. It also covers the role and scope of the dental technician in the construction of fixed restorations.

I recommend this book for all dentists and technicians who want to learn and gain experience in this technique; would that there had been guides like this when I was trying to learn implant dentistry in the mid-80s. Ultimately, this will benefit your most important person, your patient!

Dr Phil Bennett
Lyme Bay Dentistry
Lyme Regis, UK

[1] Cecilia Tomassini, Office for National Statistics, UK

Preface

"The real secret of success is enthusiasm." (Walter Percy Chrysler, automobile manufacturer, April 2, 1875 – August 18, 1940)

For almost 25 years, our practice has focused on implantology. During this period, we have seen a number of implantological treatment approaches come and go. A slightly skeptical, wait-and-see attitude to ideas that are trumpeted as revolutionary was, and still is, certainly appropriate. However, we quickly became enthusiastic about immediate restoration. And we have remained so.

There are good reasons for our enthusiasm. Using the conventional methods of implantology, patients with reduced dentition could rarely receive implants without bone augmentation. As a result, many patients chose classic restorations instead.

The approach presented in this book, involving the insertion of angled distal implants that can immediately receive a functional load, is different. With this therapeutic approach, dentists can often offer their patients individualized treatment tailored to their wishes, oral situation and financial resources.

As is the case with any number of other fundamental innovations, the history of immediate loading has been written by dentists in private practice and by practicing university professors. Such innovations arise from chance occurrences, a high level of surgical skill or a mixture of both. Brånemark's discovery of osseointegration, Schulte's call for load-free healing, Ledermann's principle of splinting, Maló's idea of angled distal implants – the list of colleagues who made valuable contributions could go on.

But however different their ideas, the reactions from their colleagues and the industry remained the same: skepticism and reserve were the milder responses with which the innovators were confronted. When the authors first presented the fast & fixed approach seven years ago, some colleagues dismissed the procedure by commenting that the dentists at Georg Bayer's practice probably could not insert implants other than at an angle.

Innovative approaches and concepts often get a cold reception by the major dental suppliers as well. Perhaps this is because research and development do not immediately sell a product and require committed investments, on more than the financial level. It takes time for developments to become marketable. And it takes partners who have the courage and stamina to professionally and appropriately implement the new concepts. It also takes trust in the developers. Listening to them, understanding their vision, collaborating with them in making corrections, changing plans and starting afresh: the willingness to do so is more often found in owner-managed small or medium-sized businesses. For the fast & fixed method, this company was Bredent in Senden, Germany. We would like to expressly thank the company for placing confidence in us and for their support with modified implant components.

Such support is crucial to success since it is impossible to completely avoid setbacks and failures. This was also true with immediate loading. The initial euphoria has abated and been replaced by a sober, scientifically founded assessment. Experienced colleagues have always greeted initial claims of treatment success with a healthy dose of skepticism. Biology cannot be "tricked". Not everything is predictable, even if many marketing departments would like to suggest otherwise.

Immediate loading on distal angled implants with a splinted superstructure has become an established therapeutic approach and is sufficiently documented in scientific studies. The function, longevity and esthetics of the restorations meet high expectations. The treatment results are generally predictable, providing that the dentist, dental technician and patient strictly observe the necessary precautions. Thanks to these facts, we have remained enthusiastic supporters of this method for years.

It is certainly not always easy to convince patients who believe that they still have a full set of good teeth that the truth is otherwise. The disclosure that their teeth are no longer worth saving and must be extracted is generally not met with immediate acceptance. At this point, it is therefore all the more important to spark the patient's enthusiasm and to offer realistic, quality solutions.

Dentists who are able to communicate this solution to patients in an understandable manner and with sincere enthusiasm are in the best position to motivate patients to choose an immediate restoration with a reduced number of implants.

If this book sparks your enthusiasm for immediate restorations with fewer implants and thereby increases your patient load, it has fulfilled its purpose.

In closing, we would like to express our thanks to our team and especially to the colleagues without whom this book could not have been written: Fabian Sigmund for collecting the follow-up examination data, Dr Freimut Vizethum for his support in analyzing the FEM examination and Dr Michael Weiss for the use of the novel digital implant planning techniques.

Landsberg am Lech, February 2011
The authors

List of authors

Primary authors
Dr Georg Bayer[1]
Dr Frank Kistler[1]
Dr Steffen Kistler[1]
Stephan Adler, dental technician[1]
Priv.-Doz. Dr Jörg Neugebauer[1,2]

Coauthors
Fabian Sigmund, dentist[1]
Dr Ing. Freimut Vizethum[3]
Dr Michael Weiss[4]

[1] Private practice for dentistry, Drs Bayer, Kistler, Elbertzhagen, and colleagues • Von-Kuhlmann-Str. 1, 86899 Landsberg am Lech • Tel: 08191 947666-0 • Fax: 08191 947666-95 • info@implantate-landsberg.de • www.implantate-landsberg.de

[2] Interdisciplinary Outpatient Department for Oral Surgery and Implantology Clinic and Outpatient Department for Oral, Maxillofacial, and Plastic Surgery at the University of Cologne • Director: Univ.-Prof. Dr Dr J. E. Zöller • Kerpener Str. 32, 50931 Cologne

[3] Am Mannaberg 7, 69231 Rauenberg • Tel: 06222 683 904-1

[4] OPUS DC dental clinic • Neue Strasse 72-74, 89073 Ulm • Tel: 0731 140160 • Fax: 0731 1401660 • info@opus-dc.de • www.opus-dc.de

Contents

1   Initial findings

A growing number of dental patients aged over 60, who are quite active but nevertheless "older," are looking for fixed, permanently functional and esthetically attractive dental restorations. However, their care is frequently complicated (Fig 1-1) by remaining teeth that are not worth saving or by fully edentulous arches with an atrophied maxilla and mandible. The complex augmentative surgeries and longer, multi-session treatments that then become necessary are frequently rejected as a result of patient anxiety about potential complications and high costs[83,193].

Based on the efforts of Paulo Maló and biomechanics expert Bob Rangert[103,104], the authors have developed an alternative implantological treatment system, the SKY fast & fixed system. This is able to accommodate patients' wishes in a streamlined treatment regimen without extensive surgery and at a reasonable

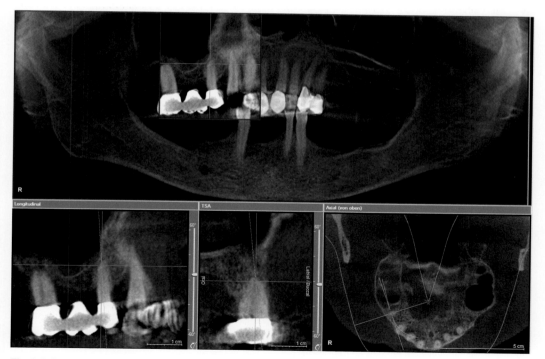

Fig 1-1 Patient with prior periodontitis and limited potential for preserving remaining teeth.

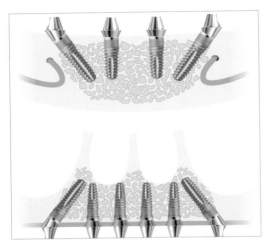

Fig 1-2 Ideal positioning of four implants in the mandible and six in the maxilla.

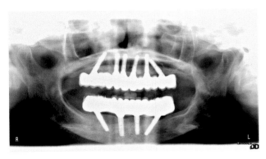

Fig 1-3 Fixed restoration on four implants in the mandible and on six implants in the maxilla.

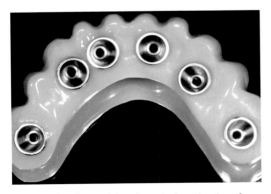

Fig 1-4 Acrylic provisional created on the day of surgery with a slight extension.

cost[89]. The surgical procedure is performed in a single session, and the patient receives a provisional fixed bridge. On the basis of the positive experience with the provisional restoration, patients often select a higher-quality design than originally planned for the definitive prosthesis (Figs 1-2 to 1-4).

1.1 SKY fast & fixed: Fixed restorations without augmentation

The beginnings of modern implantology date back to the mid-1970s. Generally speaking, patients who received implants at that time possessed a sufficient bone bed, and the implants were generally placed in the mandible, but then with increasing frequency in the maxilla[4,5,154]. Since edentulous maxillary arches are normally associated with significant caudalization of the maxillary sinus, the implants could only be placed in the infrasinus region[69]. However, such positioning of the implants was generally unsuitable for fixed restorations in the form of extension bridges; consequently, the use of removable dentures became established for the maxilla[194].

Early on, posterior support was achieved by inserting implants in the tuber region[15]. For hygiene reasons and given the large distance to the anterior implants, bar constructions were preferred in this case. However, high early failure rates for implants in the tuber region led to a departure from this technique, and in the early 1990s, sinus floor elevation and augmentation became the established procedure for preparing the maxillary implant bed[23,81,178]. Today, sinus floor elevation using bone replacement material or autologous bone is a routine procedure in the maxilla, particularly when replacing posterior teeth[47,55,141]. Depending on the residual bone height and the available augmentation material, however, this procedure requires a relatively long consolidation phase before the implants can be inserted or exposed to normal loading[58].

In recent years, the use of angled implants for anchoring fixed restorations has become established[8,91]. To enable the use of the available bone without extensive augmentative measures, however, it was necessary to develop an implant body with a microporous and hydrophilic surface specifically tailored to the high loads. Even in patients with a reduced bone bed, these implants have achieved favorable long-term results[42, 50] (Fig 1-5).

1.1.1 The concept of angled implants

The working group around Paulo Maló and biomechanics expert Bob Rangert was the first to achieve clinical success with angled implants for restorations with fixed bridges in the maxilla and mandible, whilst avoiding sinus floor elevation and nerve lateralization in the mandible[103,143]. Their publications reveal a high cumulative survival rate of 97.6%[103] and a prosthetic survival rate of 100%. They thereby demonstrated that four implants are sufficient to support a fixed bridge in the mandible and that six are adequate in the maxilla. The initial reports on angled implants showed an even higher success rate for this method after 5 years, yet the abutment and retention screws needed to be readjusted relatively frequently, since standardized components limited options in the fabrication of the prosthetic restoration[8]. Today, this problem has been overcome through the harmonized SKY fast & fixed system components[89].

By inserting the implants in the tooth-bearing alveolar process at an angle, longer implants can be used to achieve more stable biomechanical support[91]. Studies[27] have shown that one year after insertion, bone resorption at the angled implants was less than at im-

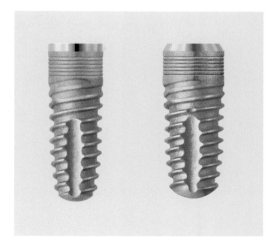

Fig 1-5 At the core of the procedure: implants 4.0 mm and 4.5 mm in diameter, ≥12 mm long with a microrough surface.

plants placed axially. A retrospective study, for instance, refuted the mechanistic idea that long-term, stable osseointegration can only be achieved and maintained under a load similar to that exerted by a natural tooth, that is, under an axial load[92]. In this study, the implants in the interforaminal region manifested an inclination of 74.3 ± 9.3 degrees as a result of the given anatomical situation. The angulation correlated with the skeletal class. The survival rate and peri-implant parameters such as bone loss, pocket depth and tooth health were not affected by the inclination. Other authors also reported on angled abutments with angles of up to 45 degrees[163]. The angle of the abutments did not influence the survival rate over the observation period of 10 years.

Long-term investigations reveal success rates of 97%[146]. Bone loss was found in 10% of the implants, at 1.2 mm on average, which again confirms that implant restorations that are stable in the long term can be achieved even without augmentative measures[146]. Ten years ago, other studies already revealed that

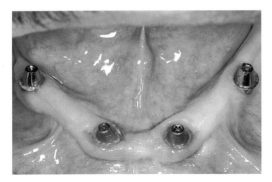

Fig 1-6 The angled implants achieve deep anterior–posterior support.

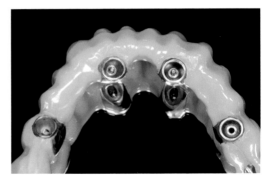

Fig 1-7 Extended support with an extension of only one premolar width.

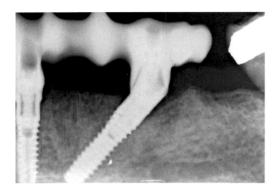

Fig 1-8 Prosthetic emergence profile posterior to the mental foramen with small loop and preserved tooth 38.

in the maxilla, the survival rates of implants with straight abutments were lower than those of implants with angled abutments. The opposite was found in the mandible. However, the authors of the study stressed that angled abutments do not per se have to reduce peri-implant stability[11,146] (Figs 1-6 to 1-8).

Several studies on the basis of the clinical work of Paulo Maló[101-104] have revealed that implants with a microporous surface are associated with a particularly high success rate. After one year of prosthetic loading, the peri-implant bone volume proved to be stable, which illustrates that this treatment approach can be successfully used both in the maxilla and mandible.

The fast & fixed approach of long-term stable support of restorations using four implants in the mandible or six in the maxilla is associated with two requirements: preventing loss of hard tissue through the loading of the bone, and enabling this optimal loading through a corresponding static distribution of the abutments. This is achieved by means of a polygonal distribution of the abutment teeth, with sufficient spacing to provide deep anterior-posterior support[84]. In patients with multiple missing teeth and the associated atrophy, this option is generally not available without preimplantological augmentative measures. However, if implants are placed at a 45 degree angle instead of vertically, the abutment penetration can be shifted to the posterior to position 5/6 (second premolar/first molar). This strategy yields broad polygonal support. In addition, the structure of the hard tissue is preserved since loading through angled implants does stabilize the bone, as confirmed by finite element method (FEM) studies[39,164,177].

1.1.2 Required features for SKY fast & fixed implants

For angulated placement, the implant must meet the associated biomechanical demands from a material-technical point of view[92]. In cases with biomechanical implant failure, histomorphological preparation revealed high bone-implant contact (BIC). The preparation showed well-developed, compact bone with small marrow spaces and without indications of absorption[140]. The high mechanical stress on the implant geometry caused the implant body to fracture but did not affect osseointegration. This clearly illustrates the importance of a stable implant-abutment connection[19,190].

For an implant to be used in the SKY fast & fixed system, it must be suitable for immediate loading. It should also feature, if possible, internal abutment geometry with minimal residual rotation and high mechanical stability. A microporous implant surface optimizes bone apposition through early osseointegration[122]. The conical-cylindrical design of the implant body and a compression thread ensure high primary stability even in weak bone, and the double thread design prevents tension and allows the implant to be reliably and quickly inserted[147] (Fig 1-9). Special abutments for the angled implants enable the prosthesis to be stably screwed in for immediate loading (Fig 1-10). Easy impression taking and bite registration allow the preparation of the temporary prosthesis for the immedi-

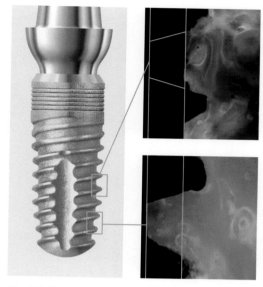

Fig 1-9 Compression thread for initial primary stability in hard and soft bone.

ate restoration. Compared to the early years of modern implantology, optimized manufacturing technologies have reduced the tolerances of the implants and implant abutments to such an extent that even high mechanical loads can be transferred to a stable implant body[20,32]. The complication rate arising from screw loosening is significantly lower in modern systems than in classic implant systems[20]. The same is true for the risk of screws loosening under extra-axial loading.

All of these aspects were taken into account in the development of the blueSKY implant system components, with which the authors were involved.

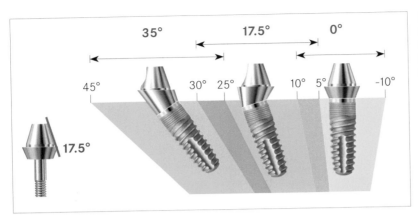

Fig 1-10 Up to 45 degrees in divergence can be compensated through a uniform outer cone.

1.1.3 Insertion as planned

Precise information about anatomical structures is required in the SKY fast & fixed therapeutic approach. By means of a three-dimensional image generated using computed tomography (CT) or digital volume tomography (DVT [also called CB-CT]), which is associated with a lower radiation dose, the residual bone can be precisely evaluated and optimally exploited for the prosthesis using a three-dimensional planning and navigation system (such as SKYplanX)[127,152]

(Fig 1-11). This software can even be used to determine the direction of insertion on the basis of the desired abutment. The obtained planning data are transmitted 1:1 to the system-compatible drilling template. Once incorporated, the latter can be used to reliably prepare the implant bed. The same technique is used to then insert the blueSKY implants. (The SKYplanX system will be described in detail in Chapter 3.) Freehand implantation is also an option for implantologists with surgical experience.

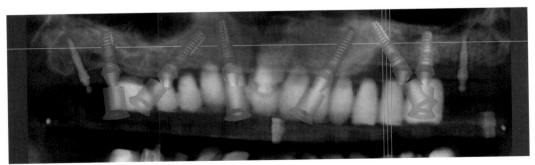

Fig 1-11 The SKY fast & fixed system also lends itself to three-dimensional planning and insertion using a drilling template.

1.1.4 Definitive abutments and immediate temporary restorations

The definitive abutments are screwed on directly after insertion. The abutments on the two distal implants should not be exchanged, even when the definitive restoration is later attached. This significantly reduces the risk of microgaps and is an important requirement for the undisturbed development of the circular soft tissue, as well as for the long-term stability of the hard tissue. In addition, this procedure saves time and money, and is less stressful on the patient.

In the next step, the temporary bridge is fabricated, followed by tension-free incorporation. The presence of a dental technician during impression taking and bite check has proven advantageous. The technician then gains a better idea of the clinical situation, which can be taken into account in the design of the temporary restoration.

Between the impression taking and incorporation of the temporary prosthesis, the patient can rest in the relaxation room. Screwed-on gingiva formers prevent swelling tissue from covering the abutment during this phase.

1.2 Older patients and their needs

Today's patients desiring to undergo implantological procedures expect their dentists to provide individually tailored prosthetic solutions that are suitable to their oral situation as well as to their social and financial status[83,193].

The SKY fast & fixed approach was specifically developed for patients with atrophy of the jaw bones who are either already edentulous or whose remaining teeth are not worth saving[67]. Given the demographic situation in Germany, this patient group is steadily growing. In only 20 years

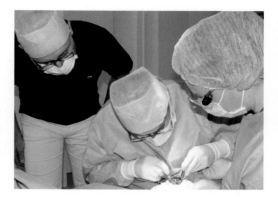

Fig 1-12 The dental technician gains an initial overview of the clinical situation when the impression and checkbite are taken.

from now, the over-60 age group will make up approximately 40% of the population, and in the next ten years, the percentage of 50 to 64-year-olds will increase from 24% to 31%. At the same time, the number of wage earners will decrease.

Currently, 65 to 74-year-olds are missing an average of 14 teeth, and more than 20% of seniors are edentulous[107]. The paradigm shift toward preventative dentistry will likely contribute to the reduction of tooth loss in adults (2.7 teeth in 2005 compared to 4.2 teeth in 1997). Nonetheless, the need for prosthetic restorations will not decrease – it will merely shift toward the older age groups. The problem is often exacerbated by existing periodontal diseases that have already been treated for years, often extensively. This scenario underscores the current and future importance of prosthetic restorations for seniors. In the future, dentists will be increasingly confronted with the wishes and expectations of patients over age 60, as well as with the associated opportunities[137,167].

Retired patients are particularly conscious of financial aspects since their income is generally fixed as a result of retirement benefits that, although at different levels, no longer offer the flexibility enjoyed by wage earners. Independent of the actual expense, the treat-

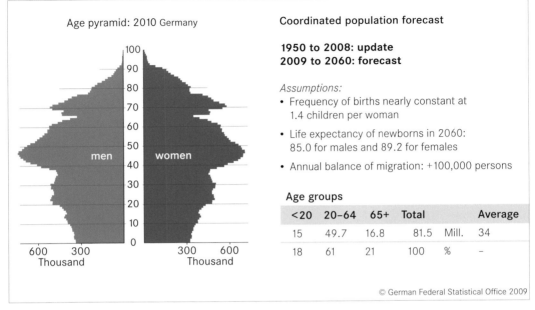

Age pyramid: 2010 Germany

Coordinated population forecast

1950 to 2008: update
2009 to 2060: forecast

Assumptions:
- Frequency of births nearly constant at 1.4 children per woman
- Life expectancy of newborns in 2060: 85.0 for males and 89.2 for females
- Annual balance of migration: +100,000 persons

Age groups

<20	20–64	65+	Total		Average
15	49.7	16.8	81.5	Mill.	34
18	61	21	100	%	–

© German Federal Statistical Office 2009

Figs 1-13 to 1-15 The aging patient clientele: a shift in age groups (source: Destatis, German Federal Statistical Office, 2009).

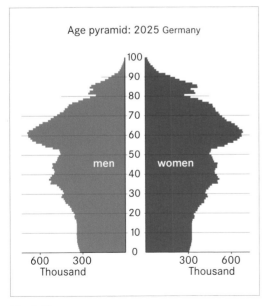

Fig 1-14

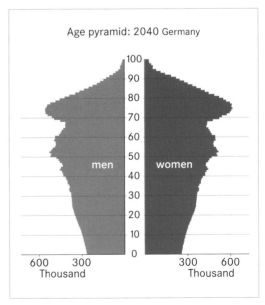

Fig 1-15

ment costs must be predictable and manageable. This sensitivity to price is associated with it a unique opportunity; however, this patient clientele is not interested in, and cannot afford, cheap, poor - quality implants. "Lasting function" is therefore the patients' legitimate demand of the restoration.

1.2.1 Quality of life from oral health

In the absence of sufficient restoration, the masticatory function of patients who are edentulous or have few remaining teeth is more or less impaired[59]. Patients who experience not only difficulties chewing and speaking but also problems such as dryness of the mouth, caries and periodontitis, tend to be even more motivated to restore the lost quality of life associated with their oral health[9,53]. Dentists can truly satisfy this desire only with fixed restorations[184]. In the initial consultation, the dentist has the opportunity to present the patient with the possible alternatives to the existing unsatisfactory situation. The SKY fast & fixed approach is an attractive option: After one day, the patient leaves the dental practice with four implants in the mandible or six implants in the maxilla that support a temporary restoration and is able to chew normally, all at a fixed cost (Fig 1-16).

Increasingly, patients need a restoration with immediate implants in the maxilla and / or mandible in cases of residual dentition that is not worth saving, a segmental restoration of only one side of the jaw or implants with peri- or preimplantation augmentation: The indications for the SKY fast & fixed method, which was developed on the basis of practical experience, coincides with the treatment needs of this growing group of patients (Figs 1-17 to 1-20).

Generally, these patients have a limited number of remaining teeth and a poor prognosis for the remaining retention elements for

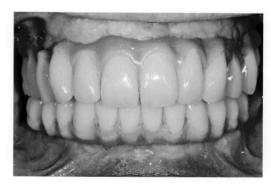

Fig 1-16 The SKY fast & fixed approach enables a fast and standardized treatment workflow with a range of prosthetic options.

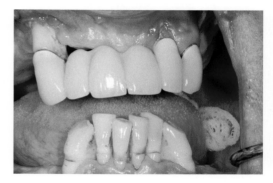

Fig 1-17 The remaining dentition is not worth saving.

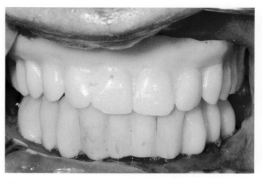

Fig 1-18 The periodontally compromised dentition can be restored in a single day using a provisional bridge as an immediate restoration.

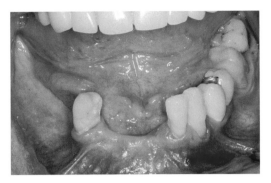

Fig 1-19 SKY fast & fixed can also be used to treat ...

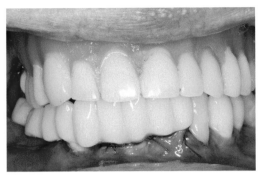

Fig 1-20 ... partially edentulous patients (temporary restoration in quadrant IV).

conventional restorations[116]. This problem can be specifically addressed in the consultation and then contrasted with the benefits of the SKY fast & fixed method. Extensive augmentation procedures, such as sinus floor elevation, postpone implant loading by several months and can rarely be combined with simultaneous immediate implantation and immediate restoration. Furthermore, such invasive procedures are increasingly rejected by both patients and dentists, not only because of the additional time and expense involved, but also because of the potential risks to the patient, particularly in cases of existing illnesses[160].

The SKY fast & fixed procedure can circumvent this problem as well. Patient morbidity is reduced, which correspondingly increases the acceptance of implant therapy[132]. In addition to the risks associated with surgery, the long treatment period involving several operations is frequently unacceptable to patients since it negatively affects their quality of life in many respects. The use of residual bone and the immediate restoration limit the surgical treatment to a single session. The dentist can therefore explicitly address the patient's individual needs, taking into account the length of treatment, risks, and financial considerations[13]. The costs can be controlled through the use of different prosthetic materials for the defini-

tive restoration – from metal frameworks with acrylic veneer, to ceramic-veneered implant bridges made of zirconium dioxide.

Hence, SKY fast & fixed is a treatment approach that is in increasing demand by an increasingly older and discerning patient clientele.

1.2.2 Determining treatment risks through a patient history

Identifying treatment risks on the basis of the patient's health status is important for ensuring the success of treatment, since general medical conditions can represent contraindications for implant-borne restorations. The patient's health status can be largely clarified by taking a careful patient history that includes specific questions on prior surgeries, medications, allergies to anesthetics or antibiotics and other health-related incidents. The American Society of Anesthesiologists (ASA) classification offers a means for rating the risk of surgical treatment[88]. The principles applying to other dental implantation procedures also apply to implantation with the SKY fast & fixed system.

The severity of illnesses, as well as the number of secondary findings and the dosage of medications, determines whether the contraindication is relative or absolute. For example, osteoporosis is not a general contraindication for implants. Treatments involving the high-dose, long-term administration of cortisone or bisphosphonate, in contrast, are associated with elevated risk[78]. Before treatment with bisphosphonate is started, it is therefore advisable to fully restore the patient's dentition and to establish above-average oral hygiene habits[162]. If relevant risk factors may be present, consulting the patient's general practitioner or a specialist can protect the patient and dentist from unnecessary risks.

The most important general medicine-related risks and contraindications include:

- chronic or drug-induced disturbances of the immune system (cortisone therapy, cytostatics)
- drugs that affect bone metabolism and may cause osteonecrosis (such as bisphosphonates)
- uncontrolled diabetes mellitus
- serious diseases of the heart, liver, kidneys or blood
- generalized connective tissue or bone marrow diseases (rheumatic diseases)
- excessive bleeding (phenprocoumon patients)
- certain mental illnesses
- serious nicotine and alcohol abuse
- untreated periodontitis.

1.2.3 Periodontitis and implants

In cases of pre-existing periodontal damage, conventionally anchored restorations can lead to overloading of the abutment teeth – resulting in bone degeneration and tooth loss. In cases where the abutment teeth have already loosened, patients feel insecure with the inadequate restoration[37,105].

In both situations, extraction of the remaining teeth and the subsequent restoration

using only a few implants, such as offered by the SKY fast & fixed system, can be a good option: Additional bone loss resulting from progressive periodontitis is averted since the set implants and fixed restoration protect the hard tissue (Figs 1-21 to 1-23).

Since periodontitis may later affect implants, successful implant therapy requires that periodontitis is effectively treated first[153]. Patients with a prior history of periodontal disease are at elevated risk of peri-implantitis, since the pathogens *Actinobacillus actinomycetemcomitans* and *Porphyromonas gingivalis* can trigger periodontitis as well as peri-implantitis[187,188]. The risk of peri-implantitis is believed to be elevated even in fully edentulous patients, likely as a result of poor oral hygiene and the remaining pathogens[153].

Therefore, patients with prior periodontal damage should receive periodontal therapy with scaling and root planing, along with regular, professional dental cleaning. If the disease is resistant to therapy, a microbiological test for specific periodontal pathogens can be performed, followed by corresponding antibiotic therapy. Likewise, it is important to encourage the patient to practice improved tooth care and oral hygiene in the long term, particularly in view of the subsequent implant care[74].

1.3 Referrals and the SKY fast & fixed system

In addition to the equipment required for treatment planning (DVT/CB-CT is the present standard), the surgical procedure associated with the SKY fast & fixed approach requires a surgically experienced dentist, to largely eliminate liability risks and offer the patient superior treatment.

With the SKY fast & fixed method, prosthodontists – in cooperation with a dental surgeon – can expand the spectrum of services offered by their practice and offer pa-

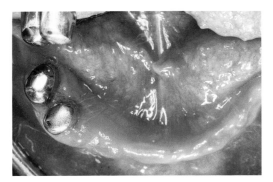

Fig 1-21 Initial clinical situation in a mandible with significant periodontal defects.

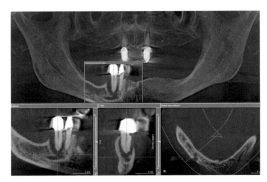

Fig 1-22 Preoperative radiograph taken before a planned tooth extraction in a patient with vertical bone loss that is no longer treatable.

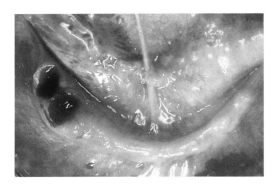

Fig 1-23 Gingival situation after extraction of the remaining dentition that was not worth saving.

tients high-quality treatment. The SKYplanX planning and navigation system serves as an interface for communication[127]. It can be used to plan the entire treatment, including the direction of insertion of the prosthesis. In addition, the SKY fast & fixed approach allows the primary care dentist to assist in or observe the surgery since only one surgical session is required. Cooperation is also easier because the SKY fast & fixed workflow can be stand-

ardized. The patient history and diagnosis are the responsibility of the primary care dentist or prosthodontist, and the prosthodontist is also responsible for prosthetic planning in close collaboration with the surgeon. The temporary restoration is fabricated at the surgeon's office or in the laboratory of the prosthodontist, where the definitive restoration is also made. The follow-up can be performed by the prosthodontist or the surgeon.

1.4 Predictable immediate restorations and immediate loading

Many of the growing number of patients with significant periodontal damage reject implants because they fear temporary, but often complete, edentulism as well as extensive augmentative measures and the limited predictability of the treatment outcome. With the SKY fast & fixed system, these patients can be predictably supplied with a fixed restoration at a fixed price within a few hours. A quickly placed restoration at predictable cost is also attractive to individuals who harbor the aforementioned reservations, or who cannot or will not go without a functional and esthetic restoration, even for a short period.

Whether or not implants can be loaded immediately essentially depends on three factors: the quality and volume of the local bone, the achievable primary stability and the exclusion of continued micromovements above 100 μm[25]. Under unfavorable conditions, lamellar bone does not form; instead, connective tissue ensheathes the implant, hindering osteogenesis.

In immediate restorations that can be immediately loaded, occlusal contact exists with the respective antagonists. When Prof. Brånemark placed the first dental implant 45 years ago, such systems were inconceivable. Advancing clinical and scientific knowledge, paired with ongoing developments and innovations in materials and methods, has led to the high quality of today's implantological restorations that can be used immediately[30,54].

The predictability of osseointegration in today's implants is primarily the result of optimized implant macro and micro design[50]. Modern brand-name implants, such as blueSKY implants, coupled with the professional expertise of the dentist yield reliable survival rates of more than 95%. If all required conditions are met, this applies to immediate loading as well as to late loading after covered healing[94,95].

This approach has yielded outstanding long-term results. Maló further developed the approach by shifting the emergence of the terminal implants to the rear through angulation. He thereby enhanced the biomechanical support of the prosthesis and, for the first time, enabled an immediate restoration with a fixed bridge instead of a removable bar-retained prosthesis.

Since implants are stabilized through direct osseointegration of the implant surface, implants lack the periodontium that natural teeth possess. Extra-axial loading therefore does not immediately mobilize the implant.

1.4.1 Primary stability, osseointegration and bone quality

Complication-free osseointegration requires implant biocompatibility as well as primary stability arising from the stable positioning of the implant in the jaw bone. Otherwise, there is a risk of fibrous ensheathment with the consequent loss of the implant. In covered healing, primary stability is not necessarily the primary concern. Matters are different, however, in case of immediate restorations and immediate loading, such as in the SKY fast & fixed approach. Avoiding continuous micromovements of the implant greater than 100 μm then becomes very important[26]. This is achieved by primary blocking through the temporary prosthesis[128].

Another significant parameter for achieving the necessary primary stability is the length of the axial or angled implants[14,26]. Initially sufficient mechanical anchoring requires a length of 12 mm or above. Primary blocking of such implants eliminates harmful micromovements.

Osseoconductive implant surfaces such as the osseo connect surface of blueSKY implants can additionally accelerate osteoneo-genesis since the formation of new bone also occurs directly along the implant surface[41]. With such contact osteogenesis, high rates of bone growth are achieved and the remodeling of woven bone into lamellar bone is acceler-ated. This provides the basis for the conversion of the mechanically achieved primary stability into biological secondary stability without any noteworthy stability gaps.

Additional parameters are the quality of the local bone and the adequate preparation of the implant bed following the surgical protocol ac-cording to the bone classes D1/D2 and D3/D4. The classes of bone differ in the amount of cortical or cancellous structure: The purely cortical bone of class D1 enables reliable me-chanical fixation; the low vascularization of this bone class limits its biological value, however. The weaker bone classes D2 and D3 do not hinder immediate loading given their higher level of vascularization as a result of the great-er cancellous bone content. Their adhesion to the implant surface is more favorable than that of bone class D1, where the anchoring is purely mechanical. Successful immediate load-ing has even been reported in very soft bone that consists almost entirely of cancellous bone structures[46,63]; however, this bone type requires special measures to achieve sufficient stabilization[108].

When the implants are immediately loaded directly after tooth extraction, the implant po-sition must be chosen carefully, so that any peri-implant defects that arise from the incon-gruence between the alveolus and the implant body are minimized, thereby eliminating peri-implant defects in the long term[29,159]. When uti-lizing the local bone apical to the alveoli, im-plants can usually be anchored with sufficient stability for immediate loading[45,149].

1.4.2 Success criteria for dental implants

Since the late 1980s, several authors have intensively investigated which factors are rel-evant to the success of implantological treat-ments[4,5,38,86,165]. They have compiled a series of criteria that need to be satisfied if implantation is to succeed. In particular, this includes the following parameters:

- biocompatible implant material
- suitable macroscopic and microscopic structure of the implant surface
- good conditions in the implant bed (blood circulation, absence of infection)
- minimally traumatic surgery
- total absence of loading during the healing process
- good prosthetic design and long-term loading
- implant is in situ
- clinical mobility may not exceed a mobility grade of 1 (DGP classification)
- the depth of the sulcus at mesial, distal, oral or buccal measuring points must not exceed 4 mm in two sequential checks
- the patient's subjective evaluation of the implant must not be less than "satisfac-tory"
- the implant may not exhibit a continuous gap wider than 0.5 mm on both sides in the radiograph
- the angular bone defect (average of two mesial and distal measurements in the radiograph) may not exceed three-tenths of the implant section that is to be placed intraossally
- absence of mechanical failures (such as fractures)
- absence of soft tissue complications
- possibility of surgical removal.

Modern implant systems are evaluated on the basis of these success criteria. The blueSKY implants satisfy all these requirements.

1.4.3 Alveolar ridge incision without significant bone loss

Particularly in the case of freehand implantation without a template (see Chapter 3, "Clinical procedure"), the access to the surgical field is created by an incision in the alveolar ridge with subsequent preparation of a mucoperiosteal flap. This allows the osseous bed, sensitive neighboring structures and, in the mandible, the mandibular nerve to be appropriately exposed for treatment. If indicated, the alveolar ridge is smoothed before preparing the cavities and inserting the implants (Figs 1-24 to 1-26).

The loss of bone by the deflection of periosteum for the full-flap preparation with the concomitant loss of local bone, as discussed in the field of periodontology, can be compensated by using an appropriate implant diameter and lateral augmentation if the available bone measures less than 1.5 mm horizontally. Fully tension-free primary wound closure can be achieved by slitting the periosteum, a practice which is frequently performed with this method. Complications such as postoperative infections and suture dehiscence are rarely observed. To ensure regeneration, it is important to slit the periosteum deeply enough to cover the lateral augmentation with intact periosteum since coverage with mucosa would cause the augmentation material to be absorbed quickly and thereby expose the surface of the implant[1].

1.4.4 Augmentation in case of bone defects

Although the SKY fast & fixed method is designed to avoid extensive bone augmentation, augmentative measures may be necessary if the alveolar ridge is reduced in a horizontal direction or in case of local bone defects. Autologous bone is considered the gold standard

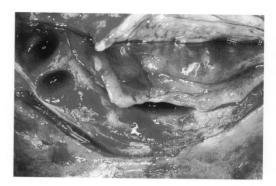

Fig 1-24 Preparation of the soft tissue reveals various defects in the alveolar ridge.

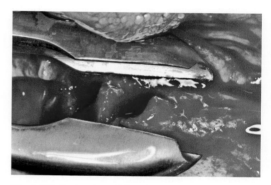

Fig 1-25 Reduction of the sharp alveolar margins in the area of the extraction alveoli.

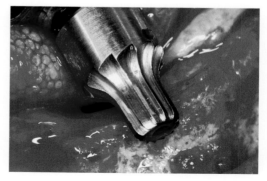

Fig 1-26 Smoothing of the alveolar ridge using the Crestotom and collection of bone chips in a second aspiration.

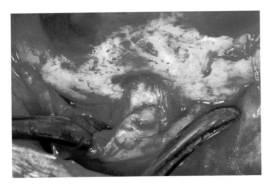

Fig 1-27 Exposure of the mandibular nerve and of the recess extending posteriorly with a radiologically monitored loop.

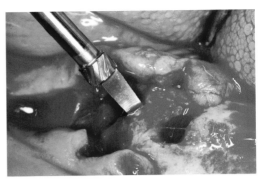

Fig 1-28 Determination of the position of a posterior implant distal to the extraction alveolus with a substantial bone defect.

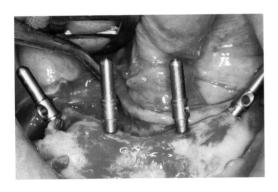

Fig 1-29 Parallel indicators for checking the axial alignment.

for filling such defects for transgingival healing with immediate restorations[120]. Autologous bone chips are generated, for example, when smoothing the alveolar ridge and when preparing cavities[6,70]. Their quality and quantity depend on the quality of the local bone, and the yield in patients with a weak bone structure is correspondingly small. In that case, bone replacement material can be used additionally or alternatively to provide volume stability and enable early ossification. Particular success has been achieved with high-collagen materials or with mixtures of hydroxylapatite (HA) and tricalcium phosphate (TCP) at a ratio of 60:40 (Figs 1-27 to 1-33).

Depending on the size of the defect, the introduced material may need to be immobilized using a membrane. In any case, it is essential for the wound closure to be absolutely free of tension to prevent suture dehiscence (Figs 1-34 and 1-35).

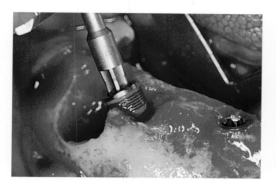

Fig 1-30 A need for augmentation is identified after insertion of the implants.

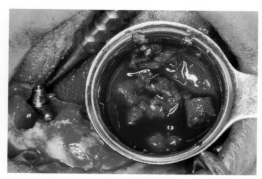

Fig 1-31 Bone chips saturated with venous blood that were collected while smoothing the alveolar ridge and preparing the implant bed.

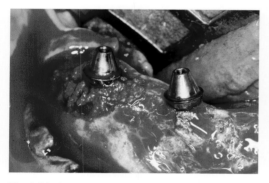

Fig 1-32 Augmentation of peri-implant defects using autologous bone.

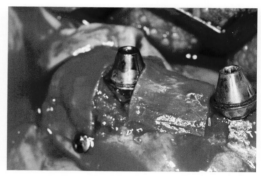

Fig 1-33 Collagen membrane vestibularly fixed over the augmentation using pins.

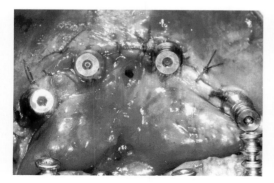

Fig 1-34 Insertion of impression posts after tension-free wound closure.

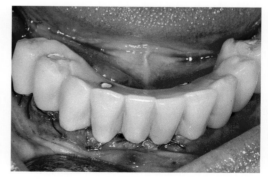

Fig. 1-35 Situation with inserted provisional restoration.

1.4.5 Prosthetic approach for initial immediate loading

Initial immediate loading requires a fairly rapid prosthetic workflow, since the temporary restoration needs to be incorporated as soon as possible and within 72 hours at the latest[176]. Manipulations after the third day can cause failure of osseointegration or lead to increased bone loss[34,176]. Particularly in view of the swelling that occurs directly after surgery, immediate restoration on the day of surgery has become the established clinical practice, since it minimizes the patient's trauma when incorporating the restoration[31]. Close coordination with the dental technician is now absolutely required, so that the temporary restoration can be fabricated within a few hours after the impression is taken. The provisional is produced more quickly and is more functional and esthetically attractive when the surgeon and dental technician collaborate smoothly. After all, the patient will wear the provisional at least until osseointegration is reached. During this period, the patient can become used to the "new" oral situation and provide the dental team with important information regarding the definitive restoration or express a desire for changes, such as regarding the tooth shape.

After the temporary restoration has been worn for 2 months, the fabrication of the definitive prosthesis can begin, guided by the patient's wishes and means[56]. Depending on the patient's financial resources, various options are available. They range from metal-reinforced acrylic bridges to partially removable veneered bridges on non-precious metal (NPM) frameworks, and full-ceramic restorations with ceramic-veneered zirconium dioxide bridges[52,135,182]. If it is necessary for lip or cheek support, the patient can alternatively receive an individually fabricated bar with bolts or attachments or (under certain circumstances) a double crown[130] (Figs 1-36 to 1-41). The different restoration options are presented in Section 3.7, "The definitive prosthesis."

1.5 Angled implants – an FEM analysis

The risk associated with the immediate loading of angled implants is determined by the loading of the prosthetic restoration during the osseointegration phase[179]. This process cannot be analyzed in vivo, however, and the results of in vitro investigations only correspond to clinical practice to a limited degree. In contrast, informative and clinically relevant results can be gathered by means of FEM analysis[15].

FEM can be used to perform complex stress calculations on virtual models. The test bodies first need to be mathematically modeled, that is, divided into calculable fields or elements that can be described with a finite number of parameters[33]. The name of the method was derived from this test setup: The calculated region is divided into a finite number of calculation fields (elements) of any preferred size. The field size of the elements can be chosen at will, but it cannot be infinite. FEM is considered a useful means of gaining informative results from virtual models of heterogeneous bodies, such as crowns, bridges or implants (Figs 1-42 and 1-43).

FEM can be used to simulate the strength of cortical and cancellous bone[186]. The occlusal load can be applied to the implant and bone using predefined forces coming from different directions. This allows a simulation of the loads on the peri-implant bone tissue, enabling the identification of potential overloading, which can cause osseointegration failure. In the same way, influences affecting immediate loading can be simulated by varying the anchoring strength in the FE model[51,138].

An FEM analysis was performed to assess the maximum stresses and strains in the area surrounding angled implants and compare them to those for conventionally inserted implants.

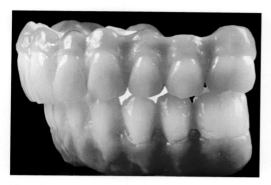

Fig 1-36 A wide range of options are available for the definitive restoration.

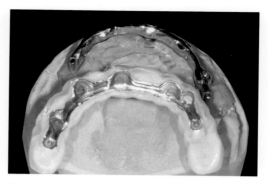

Fig 1-37 Removable bridge on individually milled bar.

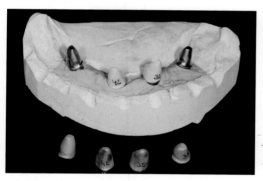

Fig 1-38 Telescopic bridge with zirconium dioxide secondary crown and gold primary crown for an esthetic extraoral appearance.

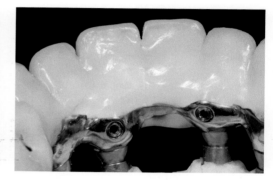

Fig 1-39 Laterally screw-retained NPM framework, veneered.

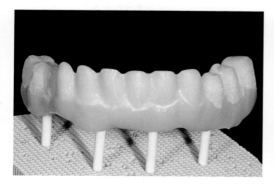

Fig 1-40 CAD/CAM-milled framework with customized ceramic veneer.

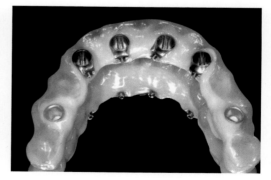

Fig 1-41 Horizontally screw-retained zirconium dioxide ceramic bridge.

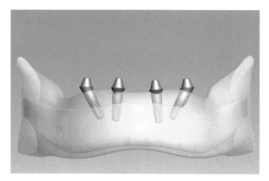

Fig 1-42 FE model with four implants in the mandible.

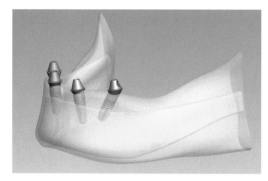

Fig 1-43 Positioning of the implants in a typical angled position in the area of the mental foramen.

1.5.1 Investigative approach

A model consisting of an edentulous mandible, implants and a superstructure was created using the FEM program Ansys 10.0 (Ansys, Canonsburg, PA, USA) to compare the influence of implant angulation and load conditions. Four implants were modeled in the bone, and the two insertion directions "straight" and "angled 45 degrees" were chosen for the distal implants (Fig 1-44). The load was applied on the superstructure 9 mm above the level of the bone. The model was segmented for calculation purposes. The modulus of elasticity values used were 106,000 MPa for the implant, 10,000 MPa for cortical bone and 700 MPa for cancellous bone. Two load situations where investigated, namely immediate loading and the loading of osseointegrated implants. To simulate the transmission of force under conditions of immediate loading, a predetermined maximum displacement of 100 μm of the implant surface was assumed at the interface with the bone under load. The resulting loading and stresses were calculated to imitate the fixation of a rigid superstructure. In a state of osseointegration, a force of 280 N was transmitted at an angle of 45 degrees to the occlusal plane, and no shifting between the bone and implant was permis-

sible in this case. The calculated results (shown in Table 1-1) were expressed as a percentage of the maximum values around the distal implant, which was either inserted vertically or at an angle. The maximum loads on the cancellous bone, cortical bone and implant were used as criteria in each case.

1.5.2 Results

Under immediate loading, there was no noteworthy difference in stress in the cancellous bone when comparing vertical and angled insertion, but angled implants exhibited greater stress in the cortical bone as well as in the implant/abutment, where stress rose from 280 to 620 N/mm². During the osseointegration phase, implant angulation was associated with a slightly increased peak stress in cancellous bone, cortical bone and implant. Figures 1-45 to 1-47 show the maximum stress levels when comparing straight and angled implants: During the immediate loading phase, the maximum stress was 14% higher in angled than in vertical implants. After osseointegration, the peak stress was up to 35% higher in the cancellous bone for angled implants. The calculated peak

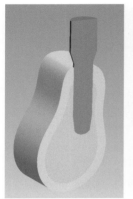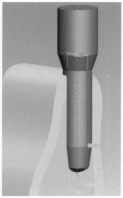

Fig 1-44 Positioning of the implants in a cortical bone and spongiosa model.

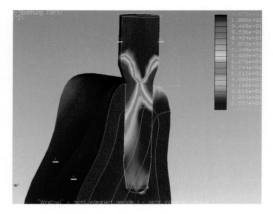

Fig 1-45 Distribution of stress in a straight, non-osseointegrated implant.

stress value in the cortical bone around angled implants was 24% higher than the corresponding value for vertical implants. The maximum strain levels were analyzed and compared with the maximum values around straight implants as well. The maximum strain values were found around angled implants and under immediate loading; in cortical and cancellous bone, they were 4% to 16% higher than for implants inserted vertically. The maximum bone strain after osseointegration in cortical and cancellous bone was 17% to 40% higher for angled implants than for vertically inserted implants.

When angled implants in a stable, rigidly blocked superstructure are subject to immediate loading, the maximum stress and strain are up to 16% higher than in vertically inserted implants, as confirmed by other authors[177]. After osseointegration is achieved, the peak stress level is up to 35% higher in cancellous bone and 24% higher in cortical bone when compared with vertically inserted implants; this situation could result in locally increased bone remodeling[128] (Table 1-1, Fig 1-48).

This analysis did not account for that potential mechanism, so the results may overestimate the effects of implant angulation on the stress exerted on the bone. If the super-

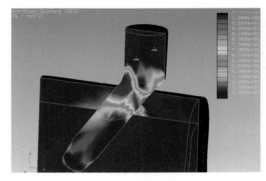

Fig 1-46 Distribution of stress in an angled, non-osseointegrated implant.

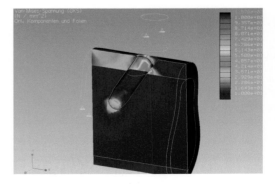

Fig 1-47 Distribution of stress in the cortical bone around the angled, non-osseointegrated implant.

Table 1-1 Results of the analysis of maximum stress and strain values around vertical and angled implants

Load situation – immediate loading (not integrated) max. displacement 100 μm				
	Stress/vertical	**Strain/vertical**	**Stress/angled**	**Strain/angled**
Cancellous bone	52 N/mm²	0.030 mm	52 N/mm²	0.035 mm
Cortical bone	99 N/mm²	0.008 mm	113 N/mm²	0.008 mm
Implant	280 N/mm²	0.002 mm	620 N/mm²	0.003 mm
Load situation – onto osseointegrated/load: 280 N; angle: 45 degrees				
	Stress/vertical	**Strain/vertical**	**Stress/angled**	**Strain/angled**
Cancellous bone	4 N/mm²	0.005 mm	5.4 N/mm²	0.007 mm
Cortical bone	98 N/mm²	0.006 mm	122 N/mm²	0.007 mm
Implant	236 N/mm²	0.002 mm	264 N/mm²	0.002 mm

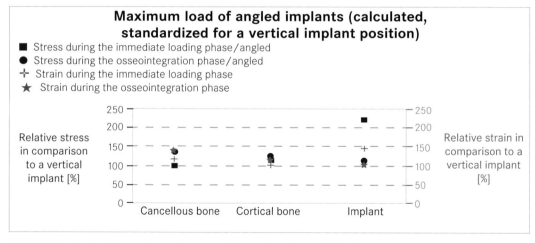

Fig 1-48 Analysis of the maximum stress and strain values for angled implants.

structure is stably fused, clinical results indicate that angled implants will undergo predictable osseointegration. The results of the FEM study confirm the importance of an even load distribution through the rigid superstructure. Particularly, the implant and the connection between implant and abutment are temporarily

– during osseointegration – subject to greater stress than they are with vertical implants. For osseointegration to be successful, the superstructure and implant components must be stable enough to correspondingly distribute forces.

1.6 Associated patient management

Apart from the cited considerations, such as the success criteria for dental implants and patient compliance, the success of treatment depends on adequate, case-specific preoperative and postoperative patient management.

1.6.1 Anesthesia

When using the SKY fast & fixed system, the entire procedure can usually be performed under conventional local anesthesia. The procedure can also be performed under outpatient general anesthesia monitored by an anesthesiologist if more extensive extractions, associated with chronic inflammation foci, are required or if the patient prefers general anesthesia (anxious patients).

1.6.2 Medications

A single preoperative dose of antibiotics can be administered to provide prophylaxis before and during the implantation, in an effort to prevent postoperative wound infection that may arise as a result of the insertion of a foreign body, the implant. The need for a repeat dose in procedures lasting several (4+) hours needs to be assessed on a case-by-case basis. Broad-spectrum antibiotics such as penicillins (penicillin, amoxicillin, ampicillin) in combination with beta-lactamase inhibitors can be used to overcome bacterial resistance to the administered antibiotics.

Patients with systemic diseases that predispose them to infections should be administered systemic antibiotics perioperatively to avoid postoperative wound infection. The same applies to patients with lateral augmentation (depending on its scope), particularly when xenogenic bone substitutes are used.

The pain experienced on the first 2 days after surgery can be appropriately treated with 400 to 2000 mg of ibuprofen.

1.6.3 Decontamination of the surgical field

To prevent postoperative problems with wound healing, the oral cavity and the facial skin must be decontaminated before surgery. For this purpose, the mouth is rinsed with a mouthwash and the perioral skin is wiped with a skin disinfectant before surgery.

After the extraction of periodontally damaged teeth, which frequently represent chronic sources of inflammation, the probability of postextraction pain and the risk of implant loss in the region of the extraction alveolus are elevated. To increase the probability of success, careful curettage and disinfection of the extraction alveolus are strongly recommended before the implantological procedure.

In antimicrobial photodynamic therapy using the HELBO® system, a photoactive dye solution is locally administered into the treated area as a photosensitizer. After a minimum incubation time of 60 seconds, during which the photosensitizer attaches to the bacterial membrane, it is activated with non-thermal light at a wavelength corresponding to the absorption spectrum of the photosensitizer (at approximately 100 mW/cm²). In the resulting photochemical process, light energy is transferred to oxygen molecules by means of electron transfer, giving rise to singlet oxygen. Singlet oxygen is a strong oxidant that immediately and irreversibly causes lethal damage to the bacterial membrane, predominantly through lipid oxidation. As a result, the extraction alveolus is photochemically decontaminated. Given its high specificity, the photosensitizer primarily adheres to bacterial membranes, so that the surrounding tissue is largely protected (Figs 1-49 to 1-52).

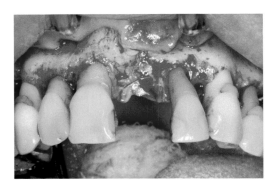

Fig 1-49 Periodontally compromised dention with chronic infections.

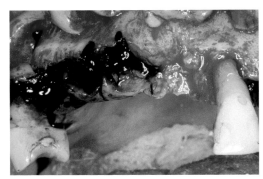

Fig 1-50 Application of photosensitizer with tamponade.

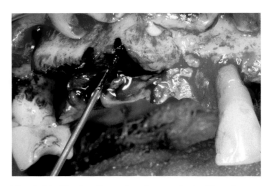

Fig 1-51 Rinsing the extraction socket with saline solution.

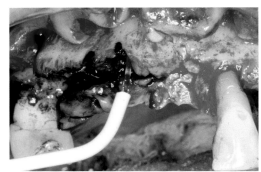

Fig 1-52 Activation of the photosensitizer using a 3D-pocket probe in the peri-implant pocket.

1.6.4 Temporary restoration

If the temporary restoration loosens or breaks, it must be immediately fixed or repaired to prevent uncontrollable shearing forces and extra-axial loads. Otherwise, this period of instability can cause long-term impairment of the implants' osseointegration process. The patient must be alerted to this fact!

1.6.5 Nutrition

To prevent the freshly inserted implants from being functionally overloaded by excessive masticatory force or local load peaks, the patient should only eat soft foods during the first 14 days (no raw carrots, breads with hard crusts, chocolate, etc.). Depending on the patient's willingness to cooperate, it may be advisable to provide the patient with another copy of the patient information documetation at the time of suture removal. In addition to avoiding milk products, alcohol, tea and coffee, patients should cease or at least drastically reduce smoking.

2   Materials and method

Implant systems for angled implants using the SKY fast & fixed method must be approved for immediate loading, and must possess an internal abutment geometry with minimal residual rotation and high mechanical stability[8,91]. Microporous implant surfaces enable optimal bone adhesion through early osseointegration, and special abutments for angled implants enable impression taking and bite registration when preparing the prosthesis for immediate restoration.

2.1   The blueSKY implant

In the early days of modern dental implantology, success was thought to only depend on the choice of bioinert material and the macroscopic enlargement of the surface area through threads or lacunas. In recent years, however, it became clear that the micromorphology and physical properties of the implant surface significantly influence the osseointegration process. Consequently, immediate loading requires the use of implants with surfaces that support the physiological process of bone healing.

Likewise, using the available bone without extensive augmentative measures requires implant bodies with surface structures that can handle the increased load. In recent years, experience with immediate loading and immediate restorations has confirmed that, in addition to a high degree of primary stability, the sur-

face conditioning of the implants is essential to implantological success. Vertically inserted implants with a blasted and etched microsurface have a high success rate in immediate restorations. The same surface processing approach can be used with angled implants in atrophied jaws as well.

The SKY fast & fixed treatment approach primarily employs blueSKY implants. These are made exclusively of cold-formed and high tensile strength grade 4 titanium (Table 2-1) and have been proven in practice for all prosthetic indications (Fig 2-1).

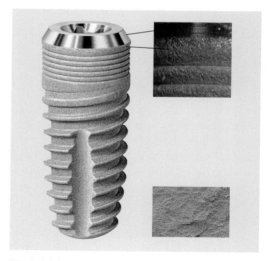

Fig 2-1 blueSKY implant with tripolar macrodesign at the implant neck and microstructured surface.

Table 2-1 Mechanical properties of different types of titanium

Titanium		Mechanical properties		
Designation	State	Tensile strength N/mm^2	0.2%-yield strength N/mm^2 min.	Fracture resistance % min.
Grade 2		345	230	20
Grade 3		450	300	18
Grade 4		550	440	15
Grade 4 cold-formed	cold-formed	800–900	> 700	> 10

2.1.1 The osseo connect implant surface

Microstructured implant surfaces are characterized by greater bone-implant contact (BIC) than smooth titanium surfaces, as well as by higher osteoblast proliferation and prostaglandin secretion[166]. The inference that these characteristics can shorten standard treatment times is supported by a high clinical success rate, as well as by experiments with immediate loading[12,28,43,45,62].

The osseo connect implant surface (ocs®) obtains its uniform microstructure and hydrophilic properties through a special combination of blasting with large particles and high-temperature etching[119]. Shortly after the first contact, the implant surface is already wetted with defect blood[50] (Fig 2-2), thereby offering osteoblasts optimal conditions for adhesion. The implant surface hence meets all the requirements for ensuring long-term stability despite a reduced bone bed. The open pores, ranging from less than 1 µm to 10 µm, are evenly distributed over the osseo connect implant surface, create an osseoconductive effect and enable new bone to grow along and in direct contact with the implant surface proceeding from the existing bone structure. The preosteoblasts migrate across the surface, adhere to the pores, differentiate into osteoblasts and secrete bone matrix[41]. Through the subsequent mineralization of the bone matrix, woven bone – which matures into lamellar bone – forms directly on the implant surface. Thanks to this effect, even implants inserted into weaker bone have a good chance of success as immediate restorations or with immediate loading – as long as all other relevant factors are also favorable[57,64,79,104,158].

The blueSKY implant features a tripolar structure in the coronal area: the coronal implant shoulder has a machined surface that is not smoothly polished and features microfine ridges. Below it is a merely etched, narrow ring of titanium that transitions into the actual blasted and high-temperature etched surface. This combination creates optimal conditions for both soft tissue and bone since the connective tissue can optimally adapt to the horizontal machined ridges, and the bone is preserved to a high level, accommodated by the microrough surface extending to just below the implant shoulder[90,106,129,170]. This positive tissue reaction is highly relevant to angulated implants since the angulation causes the implant shoulder to be largely subcrestal. In addition, the stable attachment between

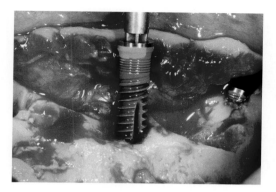

Fig 2-2 Hydrophilic osseo connect implant surface: blueSKY implant completely covered with defect blood immediately after contact with the defect.

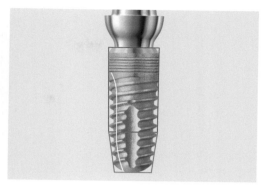

Fig 2-3 The apically narrowing implant body enables insertion in consideration of bone quality.

the gingiva and the implant attenuates the risk of pocket formation and subsequent peri-implantitis[64,157].

2.1.2 The condensing double thread and the conical-cylindrical implant shape

The thread design of the blueSKY implant fulfills two functions. As a compression thread, it enhances primary stability by compressing the bone through the larger coronal thread flanks and the conical-cylindrical core. This implant geometry allows the implant bed to be prepared in accordance with the existing bone quality[14,77]. The necessary primary stability is achieved, even in the case of slightly underdimensioned preparation in soft bone. As a result, more hard and soft tissue is preserved. The double thread requires fewer turns to insert the implant with primary stability[147]. Compression stress is thereby reduced, along with the risk of excessive compression and consequent peri-implantitis[174] (Figs 2-3 to 2-5).

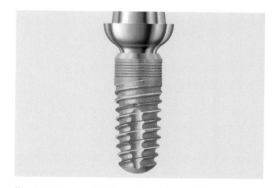

Fig 2-4 The double thread enables rapid and tension-free insertion of the implant.

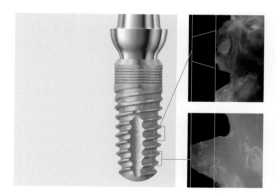

Fig 2-5 Depending on the preparation, the bone can be compressed by the compression thread.

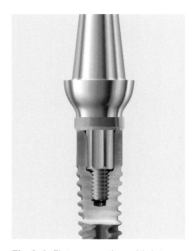

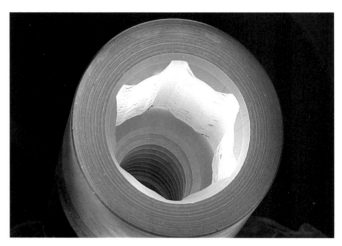

Fig 2-6 Flat connection with internal rotation locking.

Fig 2-7 Balanced distribution of force between the internal connection and implant prevents screw breakage.

2.1.3 The implant-abutment connection

For angled placement, the implant must meet the corresponding biomechanical requirements from a material-technical point of view[19]. In cases of implant failure for biomechanical reasons, histomorphological preparation has demonstrated high implant contact[139]. The preparation showed well-developed compact bone with small marrow spaces and without indications of absorption. The implant body fractured as a result of high mechanical stress on the implant structure, but osseointegration was not impaired. Therefore, angled implants require a stable connection with the abutment[139].

The blueSKY implants feature a Torx® rotation-locked, flat-to-flat internal connection. This connection is associated with two significant advantages for the prosthetic restoration: Unlike conical internal connections, the vertical height of the abutments is fixed, so they can be screwed on easily and quickly. In addition, the larger superstructures commonly used in edentulous patients are easier to incorporate without tension or the formation of gaps.

At a length of 3.5 mm, the very long tube-in-tube connection offers additional advantages[19]: The masticatory forces are optimally transmitted from the abutment to the implant, and they are evenly distributed between the internal connection and the implant[22] (Figs 2-6 and 2-7). This design therefore prevents screw fractures. Furthermore, the implant neck is free from notch stress, which is not the case in conical internal connections, where the implant neck may fracture under unfavorable conditions[65,100].

The Torx® interface has additional advantages that facilitate handling, prevent damage to the implant and ensure long-term stability by extending the life of the implant and abutment (Fig 2-8).

In the distal region of angled implants, the implant-abutment interface is subcrestal, which may result in bone remodeling. However, any bone loss arising from microgaps is very limited since the implants virtually function as a single unit as a result of the immediate integration of the abutment. In the authors' experience, the above phenomenon also does not affect survival rate.

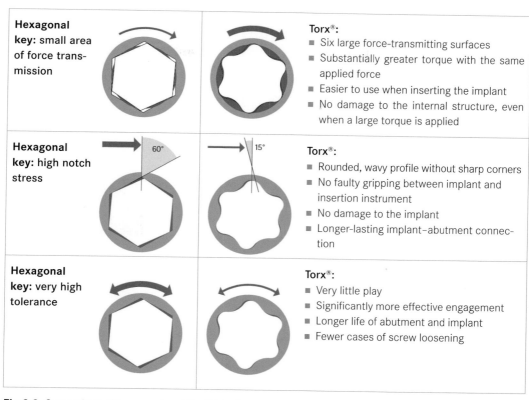

Hexagonal key: small area of force transmission	**Torx®:** ■ Six large force-transmitting surfaces ■ Substantially greater torque with the same applied force ■ Easier to use when inserting the implant ■ No damage to the internal structure, even when a large torque is applied
Hexagonal key: high notch stress	**Torx®:** ■ Rounded, wavy profile without sharp corners ■ No faulty gripping between implant and insertion instrument ■ No damage to the implant ■ Longer-lasting implant–abutment connection
Hexagonal key: very high tolerance	**Torx®:** ■ Very little play ■ Significantly more effective engagement ■ Longer life of abutment and implant ■ Fewer cases of screw loosening

Fig 2-8 Comparison of hexagonal and Torx® interfaces.

2.1.4 Implant lengths and diameters

The inserted implants must be of sufficient length (≥ 12 mm) to ensure mechanical stability and prevent micromovements of angled implants under immediate loading or after osseointegration is achieved[95,134,145,176]. This approach uses blueSKY implants 3.5 mm, 4.0 mm and 4.5 mm in diameter. Their lengths range from 8 mm (except for the 3.5 mm implant) to 16 mm (except for the 4.5 mm implant) and are available in 2 mm increments (Fig 2-9).

Regardless of the implant diameter, all three implant shapes feature the same size prosthetic SKY monoplatform. The uniform diameter of all prosthetic parts for all implant diameters simplifies immediate restorations. Intraoperatively switching to a different diameter does not affect the prepared prosthetic parts. All prosthetic options can be realized on each of the implants, using just a few parts.

2.1.5 Insertion torque

A distinction is drawn between maximum insertion torque and maximum torque strength: the former indicates the ideal Ncm at which the implants should be inserted in the bone. According to the protocol, 30 to 35 Ncm is the recommended insertion torque to achieve sufficient primary stability for blueSKY implants.

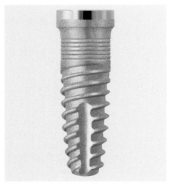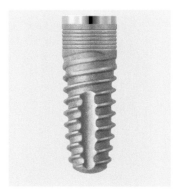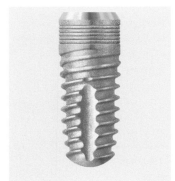

Fig 2-9 A full range of prosthetic options is available with just a few parts due to the uniform prosthetic platform for the three implant diameters.

The maximum torque strength, in contrast, indicates the Ncm at which the implants can be tightened under purely mechanical limits without damaging the connection between the implant and the abutment[20,21]. Hence, it reflects the mechanical strength of the implant. The torque strength of blueSKY implants is 198 Ncm.

Higher than recommended insertion torques may cause deformation of the bone. This may be desirable in soft bone if microfractures are to be created[114], but it is not advantageous in cortical bone, where overcompression can cause bone necrosis, as found in bone condensing[173].

2.2 Impression taking and bite registration

As long as the proper procedure is followed, a precise impression can be taken even in patients with multiple angled implants[35,72]. These studies showed no difference in the results obtained in the open and closed impression techniques[35,72]; nevertheless, the closed impression technique is recommended for immediate restorations. For the dental technician, it is important that the palate and tuber region are included in the impression. The use of a relatively flexible impression material prevents tearing or damage resulting from undercuts or angulation[131] (Figs 2-10 to 2-15). The material should feature relatively high tear resistance and relatively low Shore hardness[62]. The dental technician should be present during impression taking and the bite check to obtain a picture of the clinical situation, which can then be taken into account in the design of the provisional restoration.

In the SKY fast & fixed method, impressions for the temporary restoration are taken at the abutment level. A SKY fast & fixed impression coping is used for the closed tray and corresponding laboratory analogue.

Depending on which definitive restoration the patient desires, various abutments are offered for vertical implants, ranging in quality up to customized zirconium abutments (Fig 2-16); the abutments on the terminal implants are not exchanged. If different abutment types are combined, the impression of the distal implants is taken at the abutment level, and the impression of the middle implants is taken at the implant level.

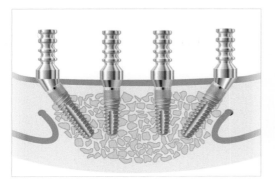

Fig 2-10 For the temporary restoration, a closed impression is taken at the abutment level.

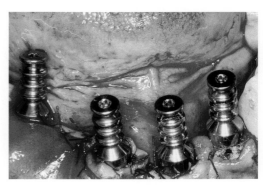

Fig 2-11 The impression copings are screwed onto the abutments with a captive screw.

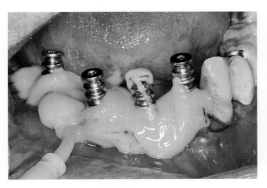

Fig 2-12 A low-viscosity impression material is first extruded around the impression copings.

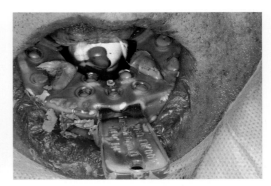

Fig 2-13 The impression is made with a closed impression tray and low-viscosity impression material.

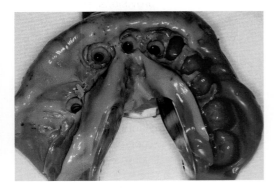

Fig 2-14 A precise impression is essential for the dental technician to produce high-quality work.

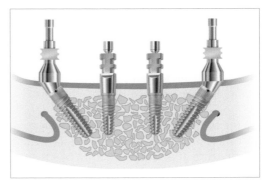

Fig 2-15 An open impression is taken if the abutments for the middle implants are exchanged for the definitive restoration. Appropriate impression copings are screwed onto the terminal abutments.

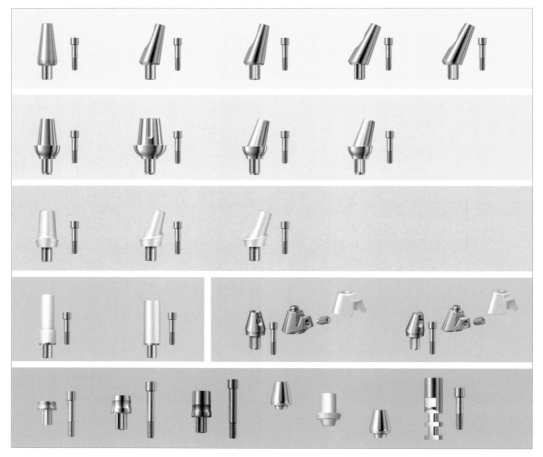

Fig 2-16 The various abutments – whether prefabricated, customizable or custom produced – enable the prosthodontist to create restorations appropriate for each patient using only a few components.

2.2.1 Soft tissue situation and "one abutment one time"

On the basis of an investigation involving two-part implants in beagles, Berglundh and Lindhe concluded that insufficient height of the peri-implant mucosa can result in damage to the biological width and subsequent bone resorption[17]. Apparently, a sufficient height of peri-implant soft tissue was not achieved by the thickening of the tissue with a coronal shift of the peri-implant mucosal margin, but rather by crestal bone resorption and the conversion of bone tissue to connective tissue.

Consequently, frequent changing of abutments is discussed as a possible cause of peri-implant bone loss as a result of damage to the biological width[10]. Inserting the definitive abutment after implantation or exposure appears to be an additional prerequisite for hard tissue stabilization.

2.3 Temporary restorations and extension bridges

The components of the blueSKY implant system enable the preoperative determination of the axial divergence between the implant body and the superstructure during the planning phase. The definitive restoration can be designed as an extension bridge – either in the mandible on four implants or in the maxilla on six implants – because bone loss and the resulting reduced anchoring surface are only found under extreme extra-axial loading once stable osseointegration has been achieved[96]. In the initial post-implantation phase, however, extra-axial loads should be avoided whenever possible since the anchoring is only mechanically and not biologically stable at this point[34]. Provisional restorations are therefore designed with only a small extension. In immediate restorations, sufficient initial mechanical stabilization is therefore even more important. This requires detailed preoperative planning and the effective intraoperative implementation[112] of the plan with critical assessment of the success criteria.

2.4 Definitive restorations

There are no restrictions on what type of definitive restoration can be used – all options are available to the prosthodontist. Although the SKY fast & fixed system is designed for screw-retained, fixed prosthetics, removable restorations can be incorporated on a bar or, given certain prerequisites, on a double crown for reasons of extraoral esthetics or patient compliance.

When fixed prosthetics are employed, the prosthodontist and dentist can avail themselves of various materials and methods, and the definitive restoration can be customized according to the patient's wishes and financial resources. If occlusally screw-retained, splinted structures such as bridges or bars are planned, the SKY fast & fixed abutments, specifically those on posterior implants, can also be used in the definitive restoration, making an abutment change unnecessary.

The range of available fixed restorations extends from economical metal-reinforced acrylic bridges to the Landsberger bridge, a new combination of metal or zirconium dioxide ceramics and composite developed by the authors that features an individualized ceramic layering technique and prefabricated acrylic veneers at an attractive price. Since the soft tissue situation may have changed since implantation, it is advisable to take a new impression and checkbite as a basis for the definitive restoration, even if the models for the temporary restoration are still on hand.

3 Clinical procedure

3.1 Surgical procedure

Dentists can choose between two clinical options: freehand implantation and template-guided implantation. For planning purposes, both methods rely on a high-quality three-dimensional radiograph for a precise representation of the anatomical relationships and structures that reflects the actual volumes (Fig 3-1). In the authors' practice, a digital volume tomography (DVT [also called CB-CT]) device is used for this purpose.

In template-guided implantology, all steps are supported by a computer and a template: from the virtual positioning of the implants in the SKYplanX planning program to the preparation of the cavity, the insertion of implants, and the placement of the prefabricated temporary restoration. The prefabricated provisional is simply adapted and screwed into place.

In freehand implantation, an incision exposes the alveolar ridge – and in the mandible, the mandibular nerve – and the positioning of the implants is then determined in a largely standardized procedure. Beginning with the vertical implants, each cavity is prepared, and the respective implant is inserted. Subsequently, an impression is taken for the provisional.

The surgical and prosthetic procedures are presented step-by-step below.

Classic implant planning is based on clinical findings and on two-dimensional panoramic tomography. In complex cases, such as in patients with periodontal disease or edentulous jaws exhibiting varying degrees of atrophy, immediate implantation may pose a prosthodontic problem, in that the surgeon may not be able to implement the implant positioning planned under prosthetic considerations as a result of the intraoperatively encountered bone condition[123].

Thanks to three-dimensional (3D) diagnostics – first achieved with computed tomography (CT) and in recent years increasingly with cone beam computed tomography (CB-CT)[109] – combined with a prosthetic waxup, the desired implant position can be planned with great predictability, in view of surgical and prosthetic considerations[123]. The 3D radiological diagnostics clarify whether augmentative measures are necessary or whether the existing local bone can be used. With immediate implantation in particular, the potential preservation of osseous structures can be evaluated preoperatively, and the size of peri-implant defects can be influenced by implant positioning[82,109].

3.2 Reliable planning through CB-CT

In dental medicine, and especially in prosthetic planning, 3D diagnostics are becoming routine, thanks to the more widespread use of CB-CT[156]. Their use in preoperative diagnostics can reduce the invasiveness of the treatment, thereby limiting the risk of surgical complications[126], which can also mean fewer postoperative complaints for the patient.

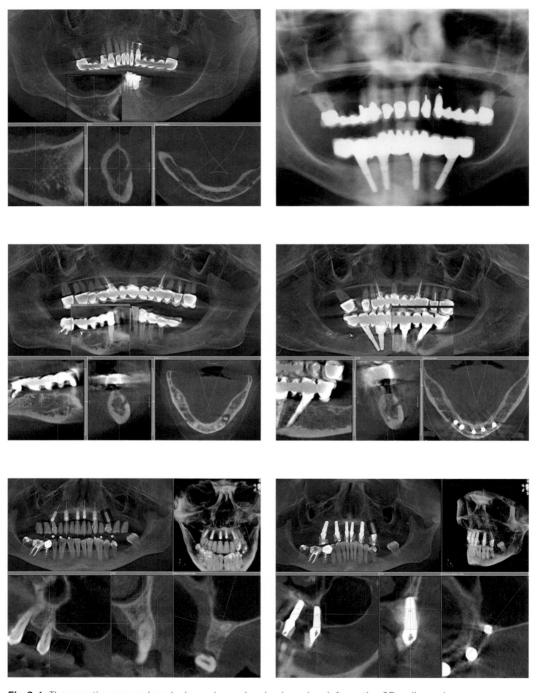

Fig 3-1 Therapeutic success largely depends on planning based on informative 3D radiographs.

For many dental issues, 3D diagnostics provide much more detailed treatment-relevant information than conventional two-dimensional imaging[111]. The detail-rich, distortion-free depiction of the precise volume of the surgical area gives dentists a far more exact spatial orientation. 3D diagnostics offer the dentist a precise representation of the available bone, thus allowing the implant position and the prosthesis to be modified such as to render augmentation unnecessary[73,150]. In the past ten years, advancements in CB-CT[113] have reduced radiation exposure when compared to medical CT[97,98], while its diagnostic value has been simultaneously enhanced[110,111].

CT does deliver 3D, true-to-detail images unobscured by overlying structures on a 1:1 scale that permit direct measurement. However, its cost, size and several-fold higher level of patient radiation exposure renders CT less suitable for the dental practice, so that CB-CT is preferred[156].

Standard indicators for CB-CT imaging in dental implantology include implants in the esthetic zone and complex situations in partially or fully edentulous jaws that require horizontal or vertical, internal or external hard tissue augmentation. Viewing the 3D image shows the treatment provider the available surgical and prosthetic options, as well as likely limitations. Depending on the preferred treatment method – freehand implantation or template-guided implantation – the procedure can be directly planned using the CB-CT, or it can be virtually planned first, using special planning software.

3.2.1 Planning using SKYplanX

The 3D planning program SKYplanX allows the use of the 3D images of the mouth and jaw (Fig 3-2) for precise information about the condition of the bone, the shape and size of the maxillary sinus and the path of the mandibular nerve. This enables precise planning of implant positions and the prosthetic restoration options[127,144].

The starting point is a diagnostic waxup, fabricated by the dental technician in coordination with the patient and dentist, that incorporates the patient's wishes and simulates the envisioned prosthetic results. After transferring the waxup to a radiopaque material, the patient is scanned with this template in place[80]. In DICOM (Digital Imaging and Communications in Medicine) format, the image data are exported into the planning program and converted[18]. In a backward planning process (planning starting from the desired final results), the optimal prosthetic implant position is then reconciled with one that is surgically feasible[71]. For this purpose, it is important to involve the dental technician in this early stage of planning and to discuss the available prosthetic restoration alternatives in consideration of the anatomical and surgical options[123].

Given this information, patient communication can be rendered more effective with the aid of the 3D image: the dentist can clearly show the patient what restoration options are available, where the potential risks lie, which wishes cannot be fulfilled as a result of the existing oral situation as well as how the restoration can be implemented[127].

Modern planning software is capable of more than enabling the selection of the implant length and diameter and virtually placing the implants in proper vertical and horizontal relationships. It can also be used to determine the angulation of the planned posterior implants in relation to the later prosthetic. A variety of display options are available to the dentist. For instance, the later abutments can be set in place, and the thickness of the mucosa or the anticipated bone quality can be estimated. In addition, the 3D data can be sliced at any location for a detailed analysis of the tissue around a planned implant. Since

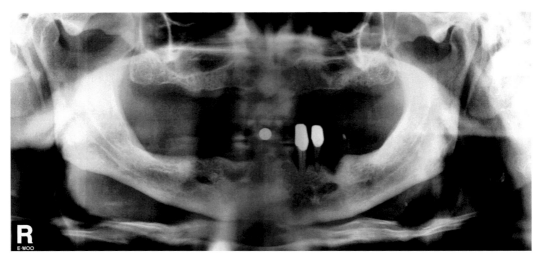

Fig 3-2 Initial situation for planning: the 3D image reveals an atrophied alveolar ridge with a large maxillary sinus.

the path of the mandibular nerve is depicted in every planning phase, the dentist can at all times visually monitor the distance between the nerve and the implant. This allows the position of the implant to be precisely predefined and translated into a surgical guide.

3.2.2 The x-ray template

The surgical guide made in the laboratory using the SKYplanX system is based on the x-ray template or the scan prosthesis that contains a system-specific or software-specific reference body, as well as the aforementioned CB-CT-based 3D radiograph of the patient with the inserted scan template. The combination of the 3D images of the crestal situation and the template with the reference body then allows the implementation of the virtual implant plan[123].

To create the scan template, the dentist first takes an impression of the patient's mouth. For edentulous patients, three miniSKY-FRP implants are inserted at fixed reference points

in the jaw at positions not affecting the prosthesis (Figs 3-3 and 3-4). These implants are used to fix the x-ray template and then the surgical guide in a precisely reproducible manner. Furthermore, they can be used to stabilize an interim prosthesis if the remaining teeth need to be prematurely extracted[192].

The impression for the master model is created using plastic impression copings placed on the miniSKY-FRP implants (Fig 3-5). After the laboratory analogues of the miniSKY implants are inserted, the impression is cast with super-hard plaster (Fig 3-6). A bite template is created on this master model, and then a centric registration is taken on the patient to define the vertical and horizontal relationships. The skull and joint-related relationships can be determined using an arbitrary facial bow. In the laboratory, the models are then mounted in the mean-value articulator using the determined relationships. Subsequently, the dental technician creates a prosthetic wax setup that already features the plastic attachments.

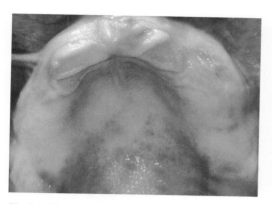

Fig 3-3 The clinical inspection revealed a stable alveolar ridge with a pronounced vestibule.

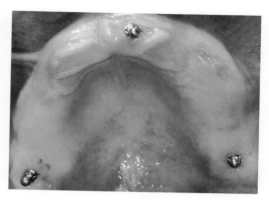

Fig 3-4 For precise planning with reproducible positions, three miniSKY-FRP implants with ball attachments were inserted at positions that would not affect the prosthesis.

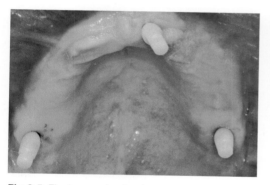

Fig 3-5 The impression for the master model is taken over mounted plastic impression copings to create a bite template and waxup.

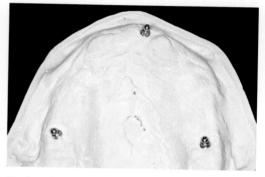

Fig 3-6 The master model with the fixed miniSKY implants as reference points.

This initial setup is tried in the patient for occlusal, articular, phonetic and esthetic considerations, and it is corrected if necessary. At the same time, the fit of the attachments on the miniSKY implants is checked (Fig 3-7).

In the laboratory, a matrix is then created on the wax setup, and the impression is injection-molded using radiopaque prosthetic material. After curing, the scanned teeth as well as the gingival margin and surface are trimmed. Through the basal contact of the acrylic teeth

with the plaster model, the thickness of the mucosa can subsequently be determined in the 3D image (Fig 3-8).

With SKYplanX, it only takes a few steps to create the scan template (two spacer matrices countered in plaster and cast) in the system-specific scan cuvette. The finished acrylic template with the radiopaque acrylic teeth is fitted to the SKYplanX reference plate (Figs 3-9 and 3-10). This plate will later function as a "zero plane": Together with the miniSKY-FRP plan-

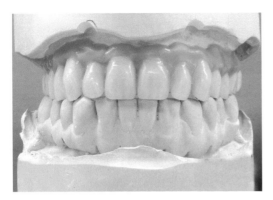

Fig 3-7 A wax prosthetic setup tried in the patient and coordinated with the patient's wishes.

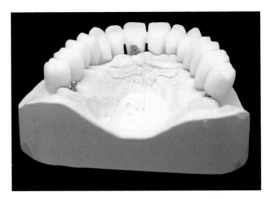

Fig 3-8 The waxup converted into barium sulfate teeth with basal contact as a model for the plastic template.

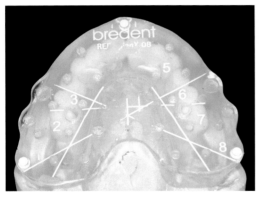

Fig 3-9 Plastic template fitted onto the SKYplanX reference plate and trimmed.

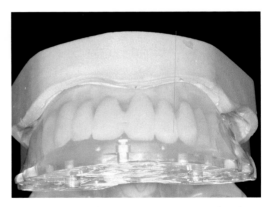

Fig 3-10 For CB-CT imaging, the scan template is intraorally affixed to the reference implants.

ning implants, it will serve as a reference for the later implant positions in the SkyplanX implant planning software and support the correct transfer of the planning data to the SKY5X transfer table. This completes the preparation for the 3D scan.

3.2.3 The surgical guide

During surgery, surgical guides aid in implementing the virtually planned implant positions. When surgical guides are created with the aid of two-dimensional radiographs, however, the prosthetically optimal implant positions can rarely be surgically implemented without problems[118]. 3D diagnostics in combination with planning programs and the option of

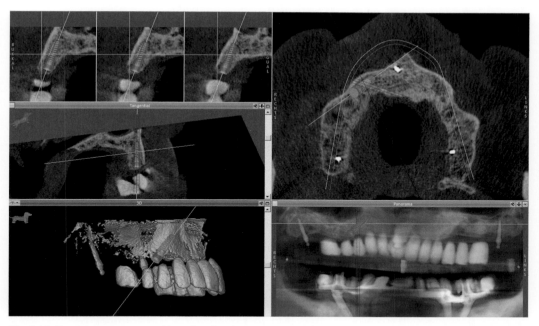

Fig 3-11 The datasets converted into the planning program provide a realistic reproduction of the intraoral situation.

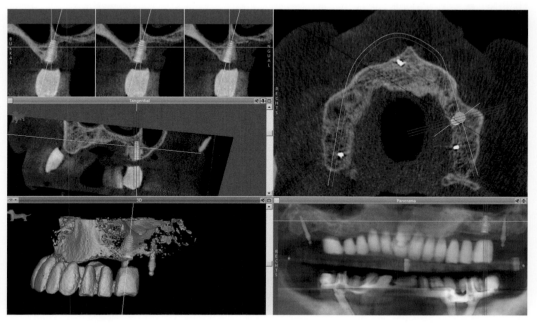

Fig 3-12 Tooth by tooth, the positions of the implants that best accommodate the prosthesis are planned according to the crestal conditions.

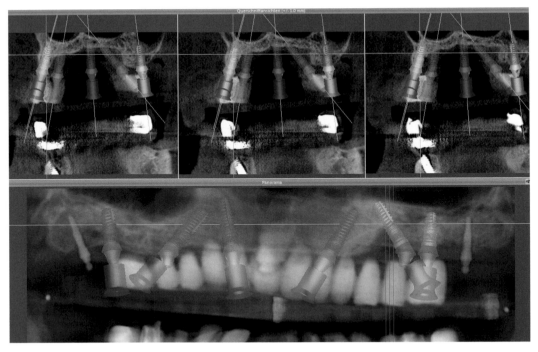

Fig 3-13 The length and alignment of the drill sleeves are specified in the planning program for the later drilling template.

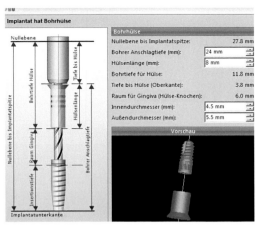

Fig 3-14 When planning the sleeves, the depth stop for the hole is defined. The sleeve length and diameter are matched with the surgical drill.

locally fabricating the surgical guide enable the precise preparation of the surgical procedure[115,123,168,189]. As a result, the laboratory can also prepare a provisional restoration with the specified implant positions before the implant is inserted for immediate restoration[93].

Transferring the virtual plan to the surgical guide involves fixing the x-ray template in the SKY5X transfer table once more using the plaster base created at the beginning. The settings are made using the planning data printed in the surgical guideplan. After the zero plane of the template is adjusted on the SKY5X transfer table, the values of the three coordinates for the x-axis, y-axis and z-axis are entered for each implant position, along with the value "depth for sleeve."

After drilling the holes for the drill sleeves to the set depth and the sleeve drill bit is no longer in use, the outer or master sleeves are bonded in place using light-curing polymer. These master sleeves can accommodate guide sleeves of different diameters, which are attached via a bayonet lock to prevent them from rotating or slipping out when drilling the implant hole. The 10-mm long sleeves can be shortened to a minimum of 6 mm as needed. After the master sleeves are polymerized in place and the correct axial angle of each drill sleeve has been checked, the surgical guide is ready (Figs 3-11 to 3-17).

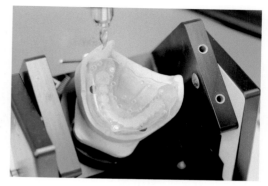

Fig 3-15 The drill holes for the master sleeves are made on the system's transfer table on the basis of the planned coordinates.

3.3 Surgical procedure

The residual teeth not worth saving are extracted, and the granulation tissue is removed completely from the extraction alveoli. Antimicrobial photodynamic therapy can be used to reduce the risk of wound healing problems.

3.3.1 Preoperative considerations

The SKY fast & fixed procedure requires that the following conditions are met:
- primary stability of the implants of at least 30 Ncm
- minimum length of inserted implants: anterior region ≥ 12 mm, posterior region 14 mm or 16 mm for an implant diameter of 4 mm
- angulation of posterior implants of at least 30 degrees
- implant positioning between the extraction alveoli, if possible (in the complete absence of granulation tissue, implant placement in the extraction alveoli is permissible)
- rapid fabrication of a stable temporary restoration
- avoidance of distal extensions for the temporary restoration.

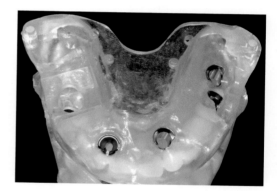

Fig 3-16 After the master sleeves are polymerized in place and the correct axial angle is checked, the surgical guide is finished.

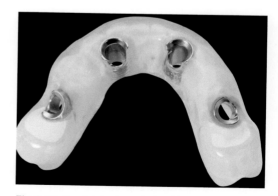

Fig 3-17 The finished surgical guide.

Fully navigated implantation takes six steps:
1.   Implant planning using the initial model (backward planning and waxup)
2.   Fabrication of the scan template
3.   Creation of the 3D scan
4.   Transfer of the 3D datasets to the scan template
5.   Conversion of the scan template (or old prosthesis) to a surgical guide
6.   Flap-free, navigated implantation using drilling sleeves

The quality of the local bone (D1 to D4) is a decisive factor in achieving primary stability. It also determines the method with which the implant bed is prepared. Bone-specific implant bed preparation has become established in recent years; in this method, the bed is intentionally underdimensioned in weaker bone[77]. Since the preparation of the implant bed influences the implant's primary stability, it is important to only use drill bits and preparation instruments that are suitable for the system (various cancellous bone drill bits, etc.) in accordance with the drilling protocol. The implants are inserted in an equicrestal position (level with the bone).

3.3.2 Template-guided implantation

In template-guided implantation, the surgical guide is first clipped onto the miniSKY-FRP implants and checked for perfect fit[192] (Fig 3-18). The first guide sleeves with a diameter of 2 mm are screwed into the master sleeves. To ensure that the drill bit is properly guided, the play between the sleeve and drill bit should be minimal. However, it should not be so small to cause abrasion or catching of the drill bit.

The positions on the template are then transferred to the jaw and hence to the actual implants using the drill sleeves and drill bits (Figs 3-19 and 3-20). With template-guided implantation, implant bed preparation and insertion are fully navigated, flapless and atraumatic (Figs 3-20 to 3-28).

3.3.3 Freehand implantation

Surgical planning is carried out using the 3D image in consideration of safety clearances from anatomical structures. The implants are positioned using the landmarks in the previously created DVT image.

3.3.4 Drilling protocol

1. The conical tip of the SKY pilot drill keeps the drill bit from slipping on the bone. At the same time, the part of the drill bit near the shaft drills out 3 mm of the cancellous bone, so that the SKY system requires few drill bits.
2. The depth and direction of the implant are set with the SKY twist drill.

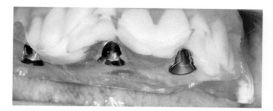

Fig 3-18 The surgical guide is clipped onto the miniSKY implants to ensure a precise seat.

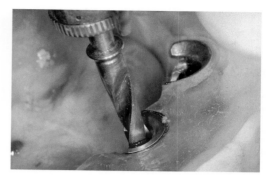

Fig 3-19 The bone quality-based preparation of the cavities is performed through the drilling sleeves in accordance with the drilling protocol.

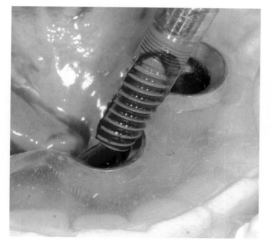

Fig 3-20 The implants are also inserted using the surgical guide; the oral slot makes it easier to insert both implants and drill bits.

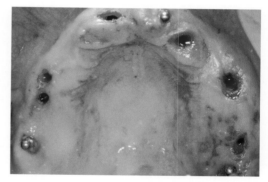

Fig 3-21 The situation immediately after removal of the surgical guide (the miniSKY implants are still in place).

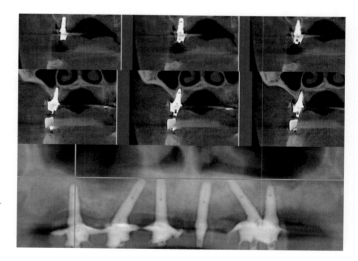

Fig 3-22 The postoperative 3D radiograph reveals the close agreement between the virtually planned implant positions and the actual positions.

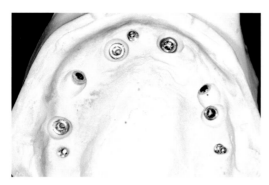

Fig 3-23 In navigated implantation, the temporary restoration can be prefabricated on the master model using the drilling template data without requiring previous impression taking.

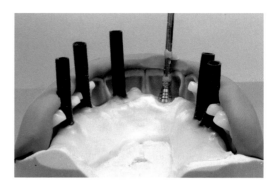

Fig 3-24 The teeth are set up with veneers using the matrix fabricated over the initial waxup.

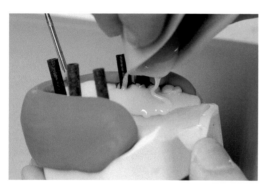

Fig 3-25 One prosthetic coping is set in polymerizing resin, and the positions of the others are kept exposed using tubes; the setup is cast using denture acrylic.

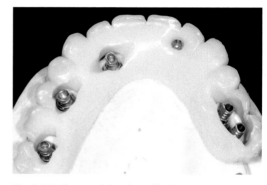

Fig 3-26 The provisional acrylic bridge with the set prosthetic coping at position 22.

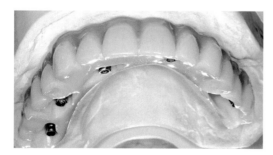

Fig 3-27 The provisional is affixed using the coping that is already in place, and the remaining copings are encased with resin in situ with passive fit.

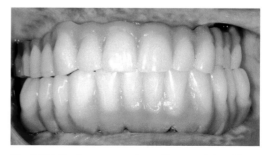

Fig 3-28 The incorporated maxillary provisional in occlusion with the definitive mandibular restoration.

3. The cavity is enlarged for the cylindrical core of the implant using appropriate drill bits corresponding to the bone quality (D3/D4 drill bits for soft and medium-hard bone, D1/D2 drill bits for hard bone).
4. Finally, the coronal part of the cavity is given a conical-cylindrical shape. In this process, no stress arises in the cortical bone. The bored hole extends approximately 0.5 mm beyond the length of the implant (Fig 3-29).

3.3.5 Surgical procedure in the mandible

The posterior support of the planned superstructure requires a stable and wide prosthetic base, extending from anterior to posterior[84]. The distal mandibular implants are therefore inserted at an angle over the mental foramen so that they emerge from the mucosa at position 05/06 rather than 03/04. This shifts the prosthetic support toward the second premolar, achieving the required broad prosthetic support[93,123] (Fig 3-30).

1. Once the midline is established, the positions of the two mesial implants are determined and the pilot holes are drilled (the distance from each of the two implants to the midline should be as equal as possible). The cavities for the two mesial implants are finalized corresponding to the bone quality, following the surgical protocol for the SKY implant system and taking into account the anatomical structures. The implants achieve primary stability after being inserted in just a few turns thanks to the double thread, so it is important to prepare the depth precisely to achieve an optimal implant position with high primary stability for immediate loading.
2, 3. The distal implants are positioned to create a polygonal shape, spaced at approxi-

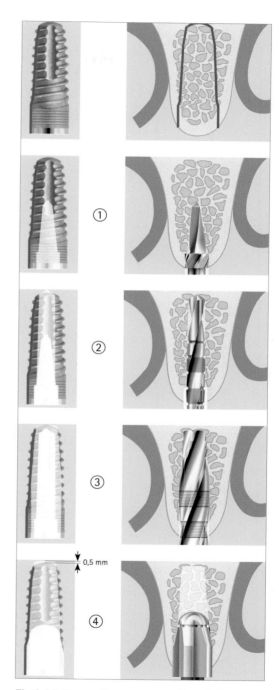

0,5 mm

Fig 3-29 The cavities are prepared in only four steps.

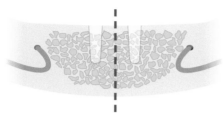

Phase 1 Identification of the mesial implant positions to the right and left of the midline; preparation of the cavities

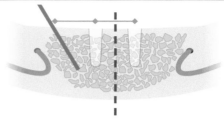

Phase 2 Pilot hole for the first distal implant; its distance from the mesial implant on the same side should correspond to the distance between the two mesial implants

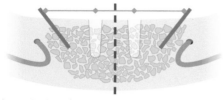

Phase 3 Use of same procedure for the second distal implant

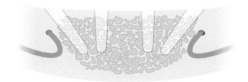

Phase 4 Preparation of the distal implant beds

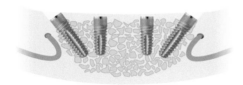

Phase 5 Insertion of the implants

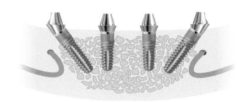

Phase 6 Attachment of the abutments

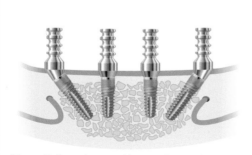

Phase 7 Screwing on of impression copings

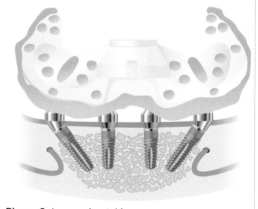

Phase 8 Impression taking

Fig 3-30 The phases of surgery in the mandible.

mately the same distance as that measured between the two mesial implants. The pilot hole is created with a twist drill (diameter: 2.25 mm).

4. The final drilling is performed as appropriate for the quality of the local bone, taking into account the location of the mandibular nerve and the path of the loop of the mental nerve[144,185]. Axial cavities can be drilled out with or without a drill stop, but no drill stop is used for angled preparation. To check the hole, an image with a gauge can be taken after drilling.

5. Each implant is then removed from its package using the insertion instrument for the ratchet or contra-angle handpiece, and it is held securely by the conical Torx® head. When screwing in the implants, it is recommended to initially limit the torque to 30 Ncm to get a feel for the primary stability of the implant[125,129]. If the set torque is reached too early, the cavity should be drilled out again, since a mere one-half turn of the implant will increase the torque by more than 10 Ncm. The mesial implant edge should be at the level of the bone.

6. After implant insertion is complete, the abutments are inserted and tightened to 25 Ncm. The straight abutments are not rotation-locked, whereas the angled abutments are indexed through the Torx® head. Should the optimal insertion direction of the angled implants not be achievable, the implants can be repositioned using the insertion instrument.

7. The impression copings for the closed impression are then manually screwed on (using a captive screw) to the abutment level. The gingiva is sutured free of tension.

8. The impression is taken.

Figures 3-31 to 3-55 illustrate the surgical procedure for the mandible using a clinical case.

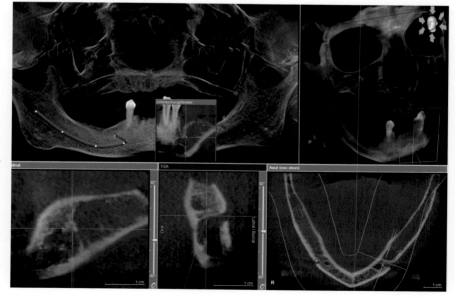

Fig 3-31 Preoperative panoramic DVT that captures the mental nerve loop (right: marked nerve, left: cross section in the area of the mental foramen).

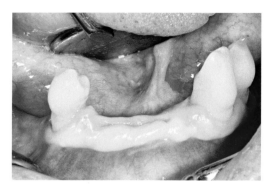

Fig 3-32 Initial situation: mandible with residual dentition not worth saving.

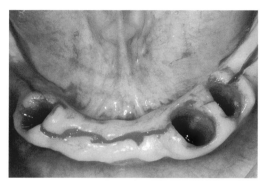

Fig 3-33 After tooth extraction and cleaning of the alveoli, an incision is made in a slightly lingual direction beyond the planned posterior implant position.

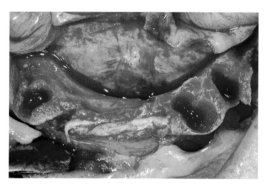

Fig 3-34 A mucoperiosteal flap is formed, and the surgical site is exposed.

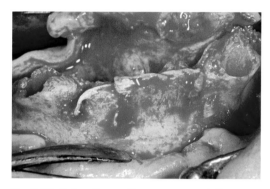

Fig 3-35 Before the cavities are prepared, the alveolar ridge is smoothed.

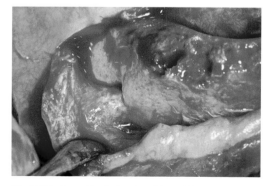

Fig 3-36 Smoothed alveolar ridge with exposed mental foramen in the fourth quadrant.

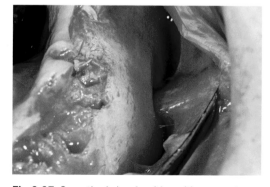

Fig 3-37 Smoothed alveolar ridge with exposed mental foramen in the third quadrant.

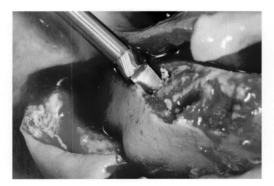

Fig 3-38 Pilot drilling for the distal implant.

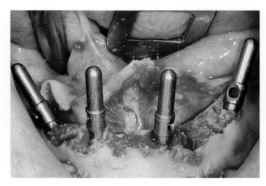

Fig 3-39 The position, alignment and axial angle of the implants are checked using the four parallel indicators.

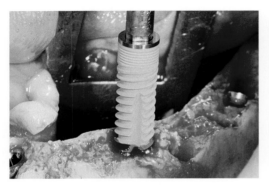

Fig 3-40 Equicrestal insertion of the mesial vertical implant at position 32.

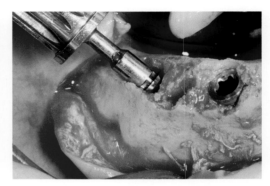

Fig 3-41 The distal implant is introduced at an angle of 45 degrees over the nerve at an insertion torque of 30–35 Ncm.

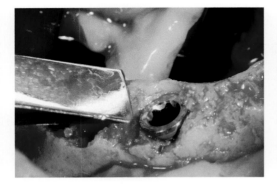

Fig 3-42 The removal of excess bone fragments to an equicrestal level also creates bone chips for filling the alveoli.

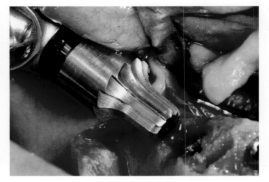

Fig 3-43 The bone margin at the distally angled implant is evened out to receive the angled abutment.

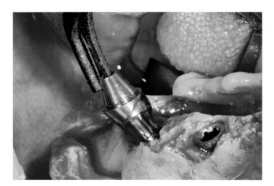

Fig 3-44 The definitive distal abutment which is Torx® rotation-locked is inserted using diamond-coated tweezers (attention: forceps and tweezers can damage the occlusal fine pitch thread).

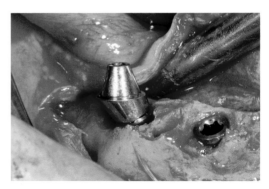

Fig 3-45 The distal abutment is in the final position; the mesial implant edges are at bone level.

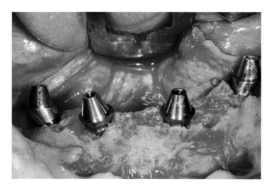

Fig 3-46 Final check of the alignment with the mounted abutments.

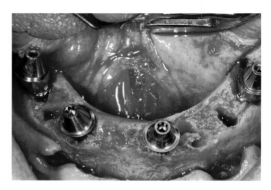

Fig 3-47 The polygonal positioning of the implants for broad prosthetic support has been achieved as planned.

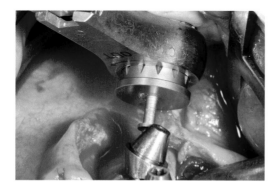

Fig 3-48 The abutment screws are tightened to 25 Ncm; in the angled abutments, the screw follows the direction of the implant.

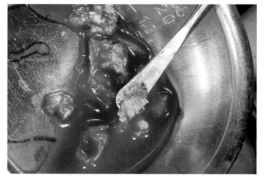

Fig 3-49 After the abutments are tightly screwed in place, the extraction alveoli are filled. Bone chips mixed with defect blood are used for this purpose.

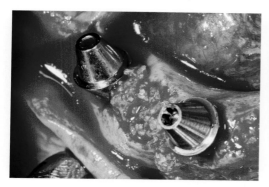

Fig 3-50 The extraction alveoli are generously filled with autologous material.

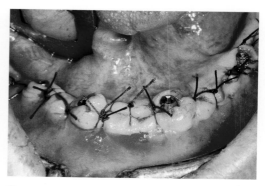

Fig 3-51 Completely tension-free wound closure prevents suture dehiscence and bacterial contamination of the augmentation site.

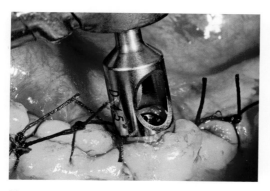

Fig 3-52 If the wound is closed before mounting the impression posts, a mucosal punch may have to be used for exposure.

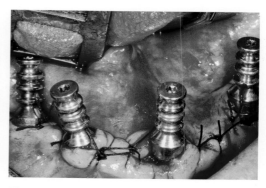

Fig 3-53 Impression copings for the checkbite and closed impression for the temporary restoration.

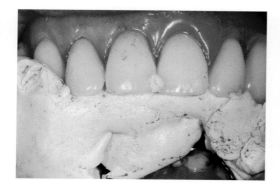

Fig 3-54 The checkbite is taken with the impression copings.

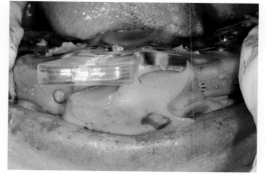

Fig 3-55 The impression for the temporary restoration is then taken using a disposable closed impression tray.

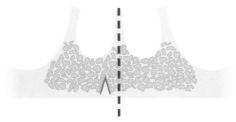

Phase 1 Establishment of the midline

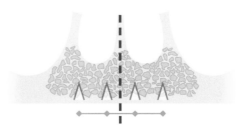

Phase 2 Positioning of the mesial implants

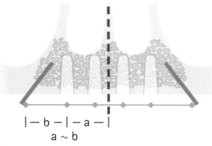

$$|-b-|-a-|$$
$$a \sim b$$

Phase 3 Preparation of the mesial cavities and positioning of the distal implants

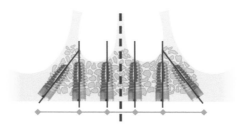

Phase 4 Insertion of the implants

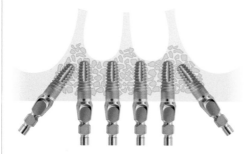

Phase 5 Attachment of the impression abutments to improve orientation

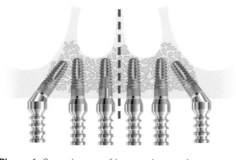

Phase 6 Screwing on of impression copings

Fig 3-56 Diagrams of the surgical phases in the maxilla.

3.3.6 Surgical procedure in the maxilla

In principle, the surgical procedure for the maxilla is the same as that used for the mandible (Fig 3-56).

1. First the midline is identified, and the position of the first mesial implant is set with the pilot drill.
2. Then the positions for the other mesial implants are marked.
3. To provide balanced polygonal support of the superstructure, the implants are spaced such that the distance between the terminal implant and the midline is twice as great as the distance between the midline and the second mesial implant.
4. Taking into account anatomical structures and bone quality, cavity preparation is completed, and the implants are inserted according to the surgical protocol for the SKY implant system. The distal implants are set at angles of between 30 degrees and 45 degrees along the anterior wall of the maxillary sinus floor, mirroring the angulation in the mandible. The orientation at the maxillary sinus follows a pilot hole based on planning and measurements or puncturing and probing. The variations in the size of the maxillary sinus must be taken into account[124].

5. The position of the Torx® head in the implant is important for the alignment of the screw channel in the 35 degree abutment, and it needs to be checked when inserting the implant (see Fig 3-57). The Torx® position is clearly identifiable at the insertion instrument. If one edge is aligned vestibularly, the screw channel is exactly vertical. In the anterior mandible, the anatomical situation can cause the screw openings to protrude labially when using the straight SKY fast & fixed abutments. To avoid this problem, 17.5 degree or 35 degree abutments can be used to shift the screw canal in an oral direction (see Fig 3-58).
6. Before the wound is sutured, the impression copings are screwed onto the abutments. After suturing, a closed-tray impression is taken. It is important to include the palate and tuber region in the impression to check the bite relation. The checkbite is also taken over the impression copings if height permits. Finally, the gingiva formers are screwed on. They prevent the swelling gingiva from covering the abutments in the interim, until the temporary restoration is incorporated. The surgical portion is completed with a follow-up orthophantomogram (OPG) or CB-CT.

Figures 3-59 to 3-70 illustrate the surgical procedure in the maxilla using a clinical case (freehand implantation).

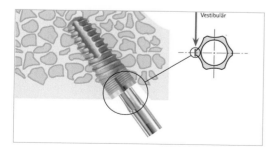

Fig 3-57 To align the screw channel of the 35 degree abutment, the position of the Torx® head in the implant must be noted.

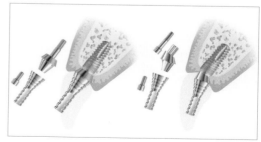

Fig 3-58 A labial exit of the screw openings is prevented by using 17.5 degree or 35 degree abutments.

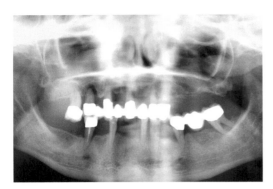

Fig 3-59 Initial situation: maxilla with residual dentition not worth saving.

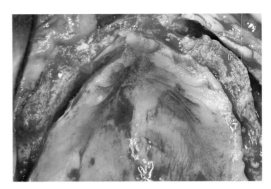

Fig 3-60 Alveolar ridge after extraction and healing.

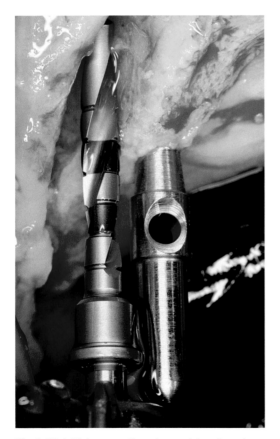

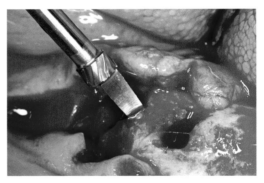

Fig 3-61 Establishment of the position of a mesial implant using a pilot drill.

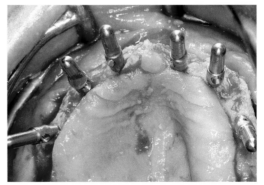

Fig 3-62 Initial preparation of a mesial cavity using a twist drill bit; the parallel indicator in the neighboring cavity provides angular orientation.

Fig 3-63 The parallel indicators show the prosthetically correct positioning and alignment of the implants.

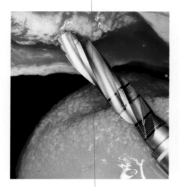

Fig 3-64 Preparation of a distal cavity without drill stop.

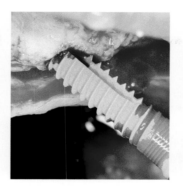

Fig 3-65 Insertion of the implant using a contra-angle handpiece.

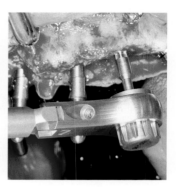

Fig 3-66 The required primary stability is achieved with an insertion torque of 30–35 Ncm.

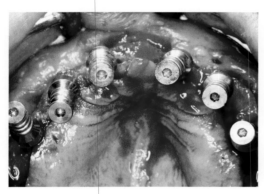

Fig 3-67 Screwed-on impression posts for checking the prosthetic insertion direction; deviation found at implant 15.

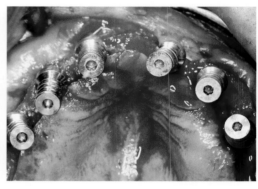

Fig 3-68 Correction of the position of the angled abutment.

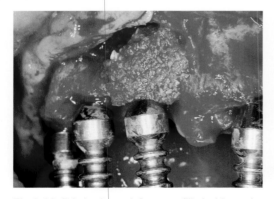

Fig 3-69 Existing bone defects are filled with autologous or synthetic bone substitute.

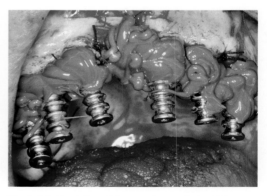

Fig 3-70 The (closed) impression and checkbite are taken over the impression copings.

3.4 Initial prosthesis

Immediate restoration with dental implants offers several advantages that are most noticeable in the total reconstruction of the entire dentition. These advantages primarily involve the patient's postoperative comfort: Immediate provisionals ensure that patients receive a functional and esthetic restoration without having to wait, and they provide the dentist and dental technician valuable information on how to fabricate the definitive prosthesis. Therefore, the provisional restoration should generally be created such as to largely correspond to the envisioned final results. This enhances the acceptance of the restoration by the patient, who will be able to grow accustomed to the future situation with the definitive restoration. Furthermore, a provisional provides an excellent means for the dentist to evaluate and check all functional and esthetic parameters at an early stage. Provisional immediate restorations thereby help to ensure reliable planning in terms of long-term stability of function and esthetics; consequently, they optimize the long-term results.

Immediate loading has become a highly accepted treatment option, particularly among fully edentulous patients[31,34,48,161]. However, patients must wear a provisional restoration for a few months so that the definitive restoration can accommodate changes in the peri-implant hard and soft tissues occurring in the period immediately following implantation as well as patient comments and requested changes. This is particularly important in patients with significant periodontal damage who receive implant-borne complete restorations.

3.5 Temporary immediate restorations

Since manipulations after the third postoperative day can either prevent osseointegration or increase bone loss[34,176], the SKY fast & fixed system is designed to offer temporary restorations that can be incorporated within a few hours after implant insertion. The fabrication options are limited since the provisional restoration must be incorporated soon after insertion of the implants. To prevent complications during the osseointegration phase, a stress-free fit must be ensured when fabricating the provisional. The dentist and dental technician must therefore develop a comprehensive and detailed plan before the procedure.

The temporary bridge is fabricated in the laboratory immediately after implantation. The presence of the dental technician during impression taking has proven to be useful for achieving optimal results. It allows the dental technician to become familiarized with the patient's oral situation, and this knowledge can be incorporated in the shape and color of even the provisional restoration.

An essential feature of the SKY fast & fixed method is the easy and reliable fabrication of the fixed temporary acrylic bridge. Taking advantage of Bredent visio.lign veneers, the dental technician can produce an individual temporary restoration without extensive preparations in just a few hours.

3.5.1 Fabrication of the temporary bridge

The individual steps involved in fabricating the bridge are the same for the maxilla and the mandible; the only difference is the number of implants.

Navigated implantation allows the provisional restoration to be prepared in the laboratory; so intraorally, only the prosthetic copings have to be attached stress-free to the otherwise complete bridge body. For this purpose, the laboratory analogues are placed in the master model using the planning data for the surgical guide. The acrylic bridge is prefabricated on this model (obtained as in the conventional procedure after impression taking).

The laboratory procedure is identical to the procedure for creating the temporary restoration after freehand implantation: The impression taken directly after surgery is disinfected, the impression abutments are repositioned in the impression and a non-hardening gingival mask is applied; finally, the impression is cast in plaster (Figs 3-71 and 3-72). To keep the bridge from exerting any pressure on the gingiva, the model must not be ground. Instead, it is important to ensure that the contact surface of the provisional is reduced and that no sharp edges extend in an oral or vestibular direction. Since the gingiva continues to swell after the impression is taken, the patient would otherwise suffer unnecessary pain. The bridge body may be slightly exposed after the swelling subsides, but this is usually well tolerated by patients, especially since it facilitates cleaning the provisional.

The plaster model is articulated using a mushbite (Fig 3-73). The articulation can be checked using the second mushbite, which was taken beforehand and includes the palate and tuber region. In the next step, the prosthetic copings are attached; these can be easily shortened if they are too tall (Fig 3-74). The visio.lign veneers are used for the setup. Since they are very thin, the veneers can be applied quickly and sufficient space can be achieved for a stable bridge body (Figs 3-75 and 3-76).

A matrix is taken of the setup (Fig 3-77). First, soft silicone is applied directly to the teeth to properly fill the approximal spaces and retain the veneers in the matrix even without adhesive. To allow the stress-free incorporation of the bridge at a later time, a prosthetic coping is placed on only one of the laboratory implants and polymerized to the bridge – in a procedure similar to the Weigl protocol[191] (Fig 3-78). Silicone tubes are placed on the remaining laboratory implants

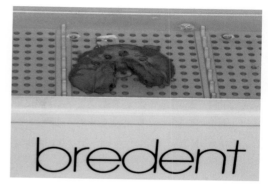

Fig 3-71 Before the laboratory starts working on the temporary restoration, the impression is disinfected.

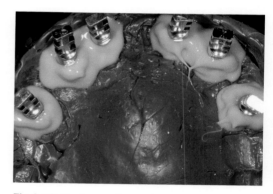

Fig 3-72 The impression copings are screwed onto the laboratory analogues and repositioned in the impression; then, the gingival mask is created.

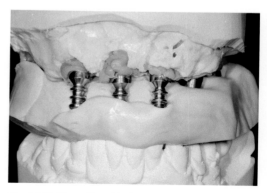

Fig 3-73 Manually guided bite registration with silicone defines the vertical dimension.

to prevent cold-cure resin from flowing onto the prosthetic copings when filling the bridge body and to leave sufficient space for their precise intraoral fixation (Fig 3-79). Once the bridge body is filled, it is polymerized in the pressure pot (Fig 3-80).

The silicone tubes can now simply be pulled off. The screw of the prosthetic coping affixed to the bridge body is loosened, and the bridge is removed from the model (Fig 3-81). Using a matrix drill bit, the space for the stress-free oral seating of the prosthetic copings is increased (Fig 3-82), and lateral grooves are ground around the prosthetic copings (Fig 3-83). This facilitates subsequent oral fixation. After the bridge is finished, all the parts are cleaned, disinfected and mounted on the model.

Since the prosthetic copings will be intraorally fixed with self-curing denture repair resin (Qu-resin), a corresponding connector is applied and light-cured around the copings (Fig 3-84). As the denture repair resin only bonds to the bridge in areas where the connector has been applied, any excess can be easily and quickly removed.

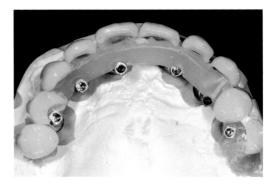

Fig 3-75 When setting up to produce a temporary restoration, the veneers are aligned from position 5 to position 5. Extensions must be avoided.

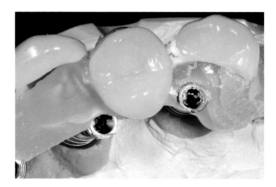

Fig 3-76 Since the veneers are thin, there is sufficient room for a stable bridge body.

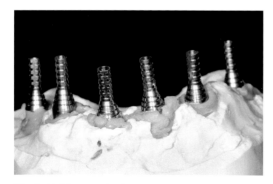

Fig 3-74 The prosthetic copings are mounted. They can be shortened if necessary.

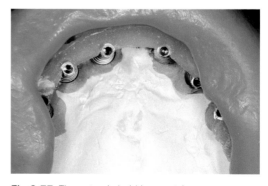

Fig 3-77 The setup is held in a matrix.

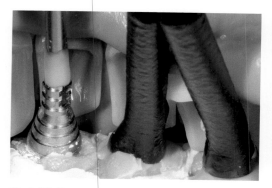

Fig 3-78 To ensure a stress-free fit, only one prosthetic coping is bonded while on the model.

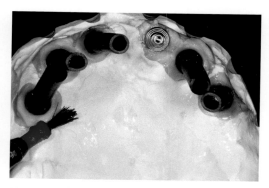

Fig 3-79 The remaining prosthetic copings are intraorally affixed with a passive fit. They are covered with tubes for protection during polymerization.

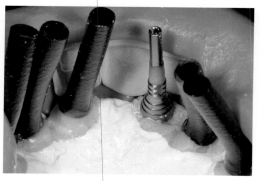

Fig 3-80 After the veneers are conditioned (sandblasted with a grit of 110 μm at 2.5 bar), the bridge body is filled and polymerized in the pressure pot.

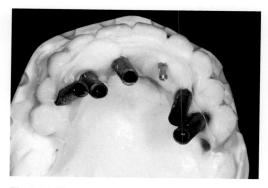

Fig 3-81 The screw of the fixed coping is removed, and the bridge is lifted off the model and finished.

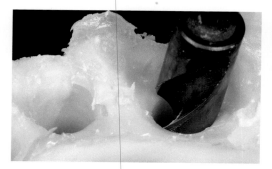

Fig 3-82 Once the placeholder tubes are removed, the space surrounding the prosthetic copings that are still to be inserted is enlarged using a matrix drill bit.

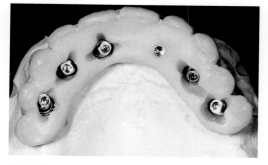

Fig 3-83 Laterally ground grooves facilitate the intraoral application of denture repair resin.

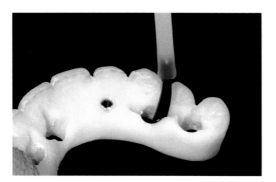

Fig 3-84 Conditioning the bridge only at the planned contact sites facilitates the removal of excess adhesive.

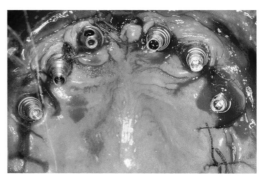

Fig 3-85 The remaining prosthetic copings are loosely placed on the abutments.

3.5.2 Incorporation of the temporary bridge

In the next step, the prosthetic copings fabricated at the office are placed on the abutments after impression copings and gingiva formers have been removed (Fig 3-85); the position for the prosthetic coping already fastened in the bridge is kept clear. The bridge is then fixed in place using the incorporated prosthetic coping. To ensure a stress-free seat, there must be no contact between the bridge body and the prosthetic copings not yet fixed in place (Fig 3-86). In addition, the peri-implant gingiva must not be compressed.

Denture repair resin is applied to the spaces around the prosthetic copings through the lateral grooves (Fig 3-87). After curing, stress-free bonding of the bridge to all of the implants is performed. After the occlusion is checked (Fig 3-88), the bridge is finished in the laboratory and polished to a high gloss (Fig 3-89).

From a surgical and periodontal perspective, all of the basal surfaces of the bridge should be convex. Ideally, hygiene channels should also be created directly mesially and distally of the prosthetic copings to enable the implants to be cleaned with an interdental brush (Figs 3-90 and 3-91).

The temporary bridge is screwed onto the abutments at 20 Ncm (Fig 3-92). These screws are carefully tightened crosswise. The screw openings are sealed using a light-curing prosthetic resin.

The provisional acrylic bridge is very comfortable to wear. It prevents implant pressure points and abnormal loading, which can arise in "riding" prostheses. A small gap resulting from the subsiding mucosal swelling is well tolerated by the patient, and lining is generally not necessary. Time-consuming revision is avoided by fabricating a temporary bridge immediately after the implants are inserted. The harmonized materials enable the dentist and dental technician to work rapidly.

On the day of surgery, the patient leaves the practice with a fixed and attractive bridge and can immediately engage in social interactions without significant limitations (Figs 3-93 to 3-95).

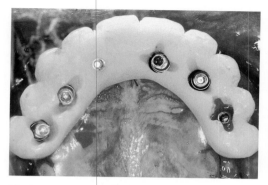

Fig 3-86 With the integrated prosthetic coping, the bridge is screwed tight. The remaining copings must not touch the bridge body.

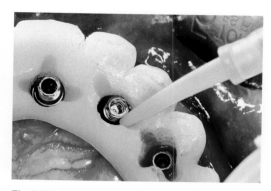

Fig 3-87 Once the contact sites are cleaned and dried, the loose prosthetic copings are affixed using denture repair resin.

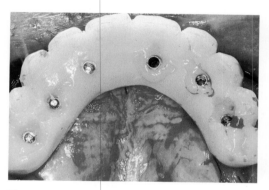

Fig 3-88 Another checkbite is taken once the resin has hardened.

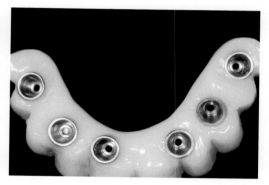

Fig 3-89 In the laboratory, existing cavities are closed and the bridge is polished to a high gloss.

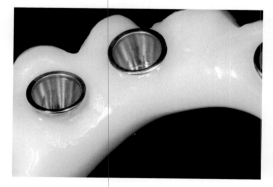

Fig 3-90 The bridge base must be convex.

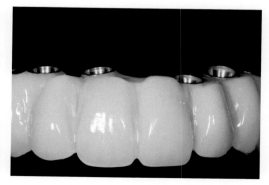

Fig 3-91 The esthetically attractive provisional for immediate restoration is ready to be incorporated.

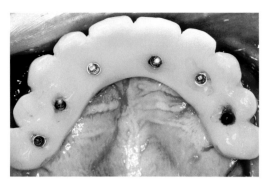

Fig 3-92 The temporary restoration is screwed onto the abutments at 20 Ncm.

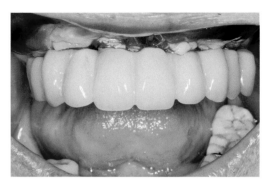

Fig 3-93 Clinical situation a few hours after implantation.

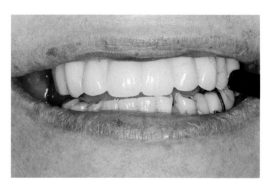

Fig 3-94 Provisional in place; implantation and placement of the restoration take place on the same day.

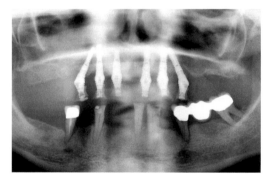

Fig 3-95 The radiograph reveals the orientation of the distal implants at the maxillary sinus.

3.6 Recall in the osseointegration phase

In addition to bone quality and primary stability, the avoidance of micromovements in the healing phase is the third decisive factor for successful immediate loading of implants[85]. In addition, the long-term success of implants depends on oral hygiene before and after therapy as well as on professional cleaning in a recall system[16].

Regular follow-up appointments are very important, particularly during the osseointegration phase. Regular clinical and radiological exams are required to identify early postoperative complications or risk factors for late complications (see Chapter 4 for complications).

The arising problems may be of biomechanical or biological origin. Postoperative early complications can significantly impair or prevent the healing process. Early complications, which can be more or less severe, primarily include the following:

- chipping of the prosthesis as a result of poorly designed occlusal surfaces or maladjusted occlusion

- fracture of the prosthesis as a result of incorrect design or bubble formation
- swelling, postoperative bleeding and bruising
- suture dehiscence following flap preparation and augmentative measures
- flap mobility as a result of inadequate fixation
- loosening or fracture of the screws resulting from tension, rocking motion or differing axial alignment
- peri-implant wound infections originating, for instance, from incompletely healed prior diseases
- pseudopocket formation in case of insufficient keratinized mucosa around the implant
- bacterial biofilm on the interface between the implant and abutment as an etiological factor for peri-implant inflammation
- sequester formation triggered by local pathogens in the oral cavity or intraoperative processes during immediate implantation
- inadequate care and oral hygiene resulting from a lack of patient compliance or faulty design of the provisional.

Implant fractures with creeping loss of hard tissue or progressive peri-implantitis tend to be late complications and can cause implant loss or require explantation despite treatment.

The follow-up interval needs to be individually determined depending on preoperative conditions and the specific postoperative situation.

3.7 The definitive prosthesis

After the provisional has been worn for at least 2 to 3 months, work on the definitive prosthetic restoration can start, depending on the specific wishes of the patient. Before beginning,

osseointegration must be checked using x-ray imaging and possibly resonance frequency analysis.

Various definitive prosthesis options are available to patients depending on their financial resources and personal wishes; these include metal-reinforced acrylic bridges, dentist-removable veneered bridges on non-precious metal (NPM) frameworks, and even full-ceramic restorations with ceramic veneered bridges made of zirconium dioxide ceramics. Alternatively, an individual bar with locks or attachments or, under certain circumstances, a telescopic crown can be fabricated and incorporated. The fabrication of these different restoration options by the dental technician is described below.

3.7.1 Metal-reinforced acrylic bridges on SKY fast & fixed abutments

With these occlusally screw-retained splinted bridges, the definitive restoration can be mounted on the same abutments as the temporary bridge, thereby reducing the cost of the implant abutments. Metal-reinforced acrylic bridges on SKY fast & fixed abutments are economically attractive restorations. Since the abutments are not exchanged, the procedure also avoids disturbing the established gingiva.

Because of the soft tissue changes, another impression (closed in this case) and bite registration should be taken, even if the models for the immediate restoration are still available. Doing so ensures the precise transfer of the current intraoral situation. Since the model is created at the abutment level, straight laboratory analogues can be used in the laboratory, regardless of the actual angulation of SKY fast & fixed abutments used with the patient. For the setup and bite check, prosthetic copings are incorporated in the acrylic base; these allow the base to be screwed in place during the intraoral try-in, thereby enabling a positionally stable examination or bite check.

Metal-reinforced acrylic bridges are economical solutions using cast NPM frameworks. The framework is waxed up around the SKY fast & fixed prosthesis copings for later bonding. Veneering involves visio.lign veneers bonded using a composite cement of the matching color. The framework is incorporated after the pink gingiva and the palatal surfaces of the anterior teeth are added and the bridge is polished to a high gloss. The attachment screws are tightened to approximately 20 Ncm. Treatment is complete once the occlusion and articulation are checked and the patient has been instructed in the available cleaning options, using small brushes and super floss.

Figures 3-96 to 3-110 illustrate the procedure using a clinical case.

3.7.2 Customized restoration options with the SKY abutment line

The SKY fast & fixed system is designed for primary splinted constructions and therefore does not offer any protection against rotation in the individual positions. A combination with non-rotating SKY abutments requires an impression to be taken at the implant level for the corresponding implants. For the definitive restoration, the option of combining SKY abutments with SKY fast & fixed abutments on the angled implants is always available.

When the impression is taken, the SKY fast & fixed abutments remain in the mouth at a 35 degree angle, whereas the abutments for the temporary restoration on the mesial implants are removed. Hence, the impression is taken at the abutment level for the angled implants and at the implant level for the axially inserted implants. SKY open-tray impression abutments are screwed onto the mesial implants, ensuring the transfer of the precise

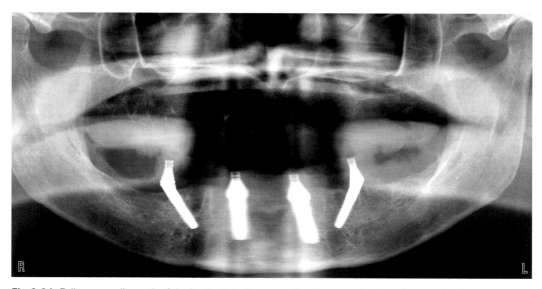

Fig 3-96 Follow-up radiograph of the implants before removing the superstructure for examination purposes.

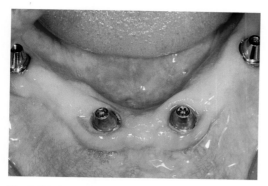

Fig 3-97 A new impression is taken for the definitive restoration in view of the changes in the soft tissue.

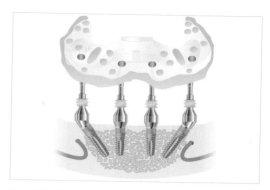

Fig 3-98 Without changing the abutments of the temporary restoration, the open-tray impression copings are screwed on at approximately 10 Ncm.

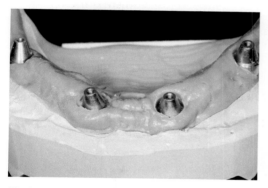

Fig 3-99 Straight laboratory analogues are used for the model, regardless of the intraoral situation.

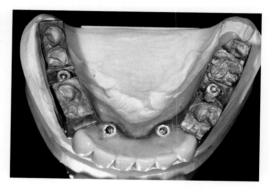

Fig 3-100 The plastic base for the setup and bite check can be securely screwed on thanks to the integrated prosthetic copings.

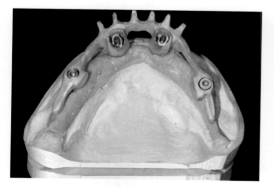

Fig 3-101 Fabrication of an NPM framework to receive the acrylic facing with prefabricated veneers.

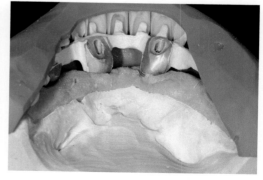

Fig 3-102 The veneers are aligned on the matrix.

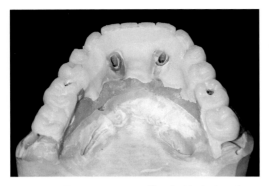

Fig 3-103 The veneers are affixed with dual-curing composite cement.

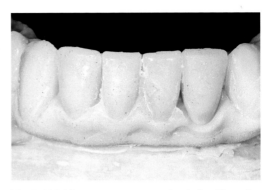

Fig 3-104 The veneers are completely fixed in resin to the gingiva.

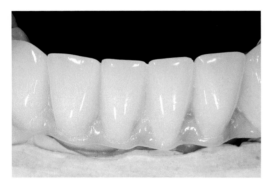

Fig 3-105 The bridge is modified with gingiva-like resin, and the contact surface is reduced.

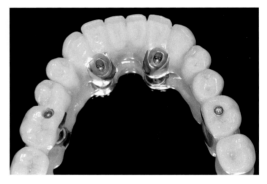

Fig 3-106 The cast NPM framework veneered with acrylic is finished.

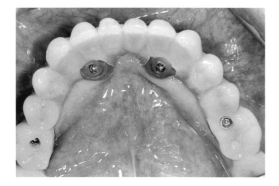

Fig 3-107 The prosthetic copings can be fixed in vitro or in vivo at the time the superstructure is incorporated.

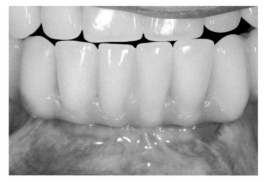

Fig 3-108 The finished definitive restoration after incorporation, during occlusion check.

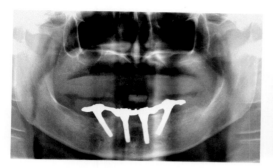

Fig 3-109 Follow-up radiograph after incorporation of the prosthesis to determine the peri-implant bone level.

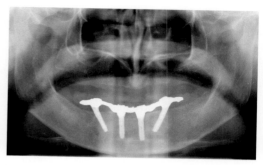

Fig 3-110 Follow-up radiograph after one year with no evidence of changes in the peri-implant bone level.

Torx® position. SKY fast & fixed open-tray impression copings are screwed onto the 35 degree abutments. After the model is created, the corresponding SKY fast & fixed prosthetic copings without rotation lock or the Torx® rotation-locked SKY abutments are selected.

3.7.3 Dentist-removable bridges with customized lateral screw connection, NPM framework and visio.lign veneers

The advantage of dentist-removable bridges is that they can generally be removed without complications for professional cleaning. In addition, the bridge can be fastened with screws or bolts; this is helpful for all implant-borne bridges since it allows them to be removed and modified if necessary.

To produce a dentist-removable bridge, the bite registration and individual tray are first prepared using an initial model created using an alginate impression. For bite registration, a plastic base plate is affixed to the two terminal SKY fast & fixed abutments. In the mouth, the prosthetic is supported by bone rather than the mucosa. An anterior setup provides an initial idea of the esthetics.

An open impression is taken on SKY impression abutments and SKY fast & fixed impression copings that have already been splinted in the laboratory using a resin bar. To counter the shrinkage of the resin, the connections must be separated again after complete polymerization. This is done by means of thin cuts corresponding to the number of pontics (identifying the positions helps to prevent errors). After using dental floss to ensure that there are no undesired contact areas, the individual elements are intraorally splinted with a minimal amount of resin. The open impression is taken with a customized or laboratory-made custom tray. The SKY impression abutments and the SKY fast & fixed impression copings are splinted in the impression. The model analogues should always be held with forceps while being screwed on to prevent the impression abutments from rotating in the impression. The master model is prepared using the described procedure. The choice of a hard or soft gingival mask depends on the planned restoration and the method chosen by the dental technician.

The setup is created using visio.lign veneers. The patient can preview the final results of the new fixed bridge restoration in an esthetic try-in with the visio.lign veneers. A silicone matrix is created beforehand for the setup. The matrix is made of two silicone phases to precisely reproduce the interdental spaces and ensure a secure hold of the veneer shells in the matrix. As a first layer, a soft silicone (55 Shore) that reproduces fine detail is directly applied to the setup using the extruder gun. Haptosil (90 Shore) is used for the second layer, giving the matrix the required stability.

For the visio.lign bridge with NPM framework, SKY "esthetic line" abutments are used in the anterior region. The matrix reveals the bridge's dimensions and verifies the abutment selection. Divergence of the SKY fast & fixed prosthetic copings can be compensated by an appropriate outer cone, for instance. The framework is then waxed up while frequently checking against the matrix. Spruing, investing and casting follows the Bredent casting technique developed by Andreas Sabath. After finishing, the stress-free fit of the framework on the abutments must be ensured (passive fit). Lateral screws can then be screwed in hand-tight without using great force.

The framework is then conditioned, and opaquer is applied. After they are cleaned, the visio.lign veneers are blasted using 110-μm blasting abrasive at 2.5 bar, and the resulting dust is removed using oil-free compressed air. Steam blasting, on the other hand, would leave a moisture residue and negatively affect bonding. A bonding agent must be applied. The veneers are bonded to the bridge framework using composite cement. They are customized using composite.

The abutment screws are tightened to 25 Ncm for this type of restoration. Then, the articulation and occlusion are checked as well as the restoration's suitability for cleaning with small brushes and super floss. Finally, the patient receives detailed instructions on maintaining the bridge's hygiene.

Figures 3-111 to 3-150 depict a clinical example of restoration with dentist-removable bridges.

3.7.4 The Landsberger bridge

The so-called Landsberger bridge is a dentist-removable zirconium dioxide bridge developed by the authors that features a prefabricated horizontal screw attachment, a universal connecting element abutment, a zirconium dioxide framework, ceramic veneers in the anterior region and visio.lign veneers in the posterior region. The combination of these materials with the fast & fixed treatment approach yields a restoration that is both economical and esthetically attractive. In addition, there are significant advantages associated with the use of zirconium dioxide as the framework material.

In total prostheses, the vertical loss of bone and soft tissue structures is frequently very large, and the length of the anterior teeth should not exceed 11 mm. Therefore, the design of the pink/white esthetics with a pink gingival portion is essential to the success of such a bridge. In the past, the drawbacks of these restorations were their weight and the distortion of the (metal) frameworks, but the relatively light, distortion-free biocompatible zirconium dioxide is now used as a versatile alternative material.

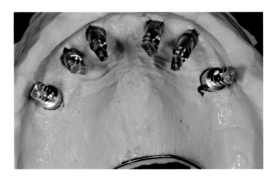

Fig 3-111 If standard abutments cannot be used as a result of the alignment of the mesial implants, a closed impression is first taken to produce an initial model.

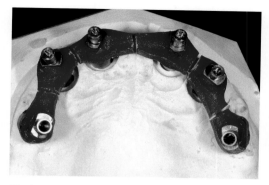

Fig 3-112 Blocking compound is used on the initial model to create a blocked out plastic bar as a test piece...

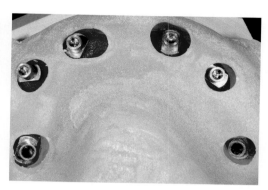

Fig 3-113 ...and a custom tray is created on top; then, the bar is separated again.

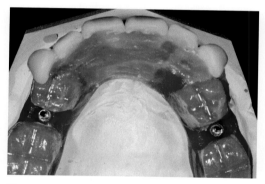

Fig 3-114 The setup is stably fixed in place over the distal implants for a bite check and an esthetic try-in.

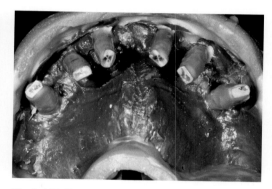

Fig 3-115 The repositioned model analogues are embedded in wax to create the gingival mask when taking the definitive impression.

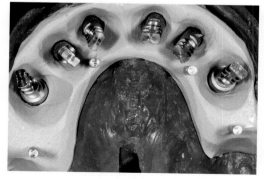

Fig 3-116 The gingival mask of hard plastic is finished, the model analogues are repositioned and a plaster model is created.

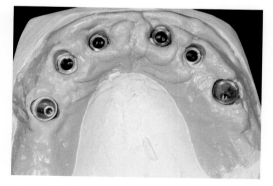

Figs 3-117 The two terminal analogues are at the abutment level and the mesial analogues are at the implant level.

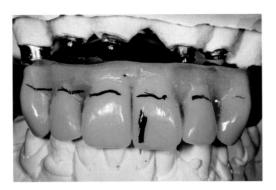

Fig 3-118 The individualized setup incorporating the corrections from the try-in is repositioned on the model base without the gingival mask.

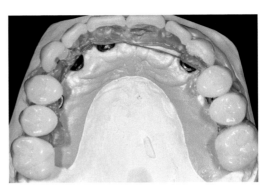

Fig 3-119 The final setup is created with veneers.

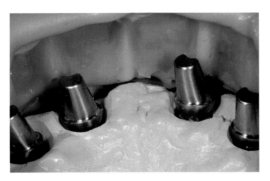

Fig 3-120 Using the two-layer matrix taken over the set-up, the abutments for the anterior region are selected (in this case, rotation-locked SKY esthetic abutments angled at 15 degrees were chosen because of the alignment).

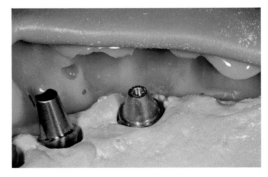

Fig 3-121 Distally, a deviation can be compensated by a 17.5 degree outer cone.

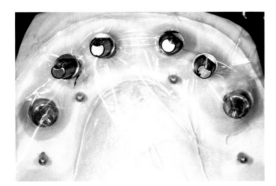

Fig 3-122 The model is protected with cellophane film before individually grinding the titanium abutments to correspond to the matrix.

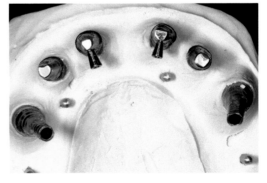

Fig 3-123 A horizontal screw connection is used for the two mesial abutments.

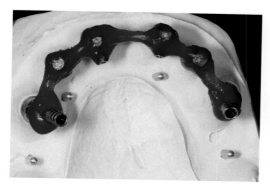

Fig 3-124 After blocking out the screw channels, the framework is modeled step-by-step with burnout plastic to prevent contraction stress.

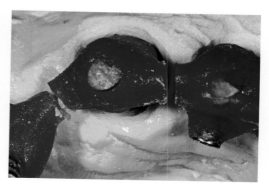

Fig 3-125 The model is cut and left to sit overnight: The resulting reduction of residual monomers improves the casting and fit.

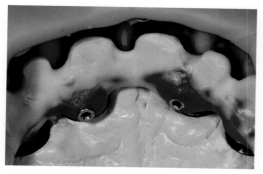

Fig 3-126 The next day, the framework is completely modeled with continuous reference to the matrix.

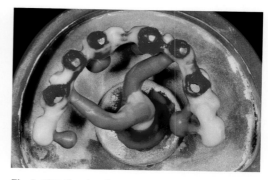

Fig 3-127 Spruing, investing and casting according to the Sabath technique...

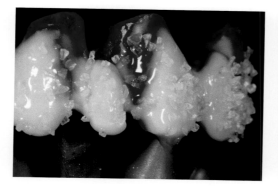

Fig 3-128 ...with burnout retention aids also being applied.

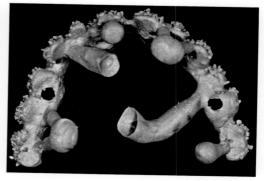

Fig 3-129 By precisely weighing the wax, the casting can be done in a vacuum pressure casting procedure without a button, thus avoiding contraction stress.

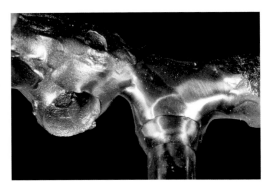

Fig 3-130 The cast framework is finished, and the prosthetic copings are adhered after being conditioned.

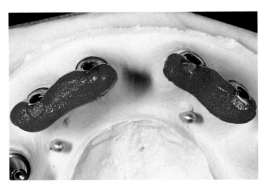

Fig 3-131 An insertion key is created for precise abutment positioning.

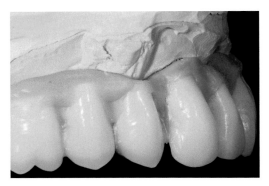

Fig 3-132 For a final esthetic try-in, the veneers are affixed to the framework using esthetic wax.

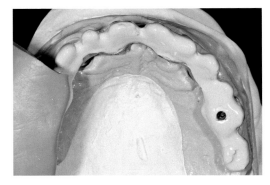

Fig 3-133 Opaquer and conditioner are applied to the framework, and bonding agent is applied to the veneers.

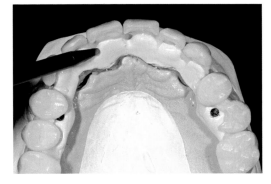

Fig 3-134 The veneers are fixed in place using dual-curing composite cement.

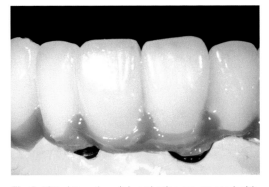

Fig 3-135 Attractive pink esthetics are created with the corresponding materials.

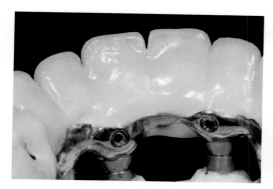

Fig 3-136 The finished and polished restoration can now be incorporated.

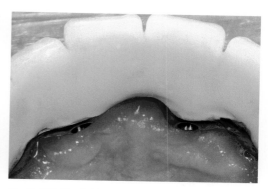

Fig 3-137 The bridge is tightened on the abutments at 25 Ncm, and the lateral screws are hand-tightened.

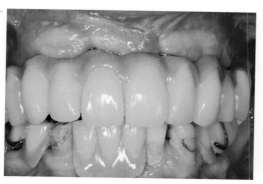

Fig 3-138 The patient asked for a predictable, esthetic result, and her wishes were met.

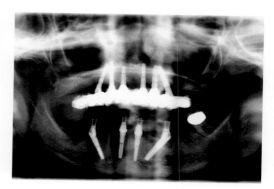

Fig 3-139 Follow-up radiograph of the prosthetic restoration in the maxilla after additional immediate implantation and restoration in the mandible.

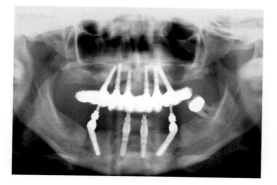

Fig 3-140 Radiological follow-up of the implants with immediate restoration before the final prosthetic restoration.

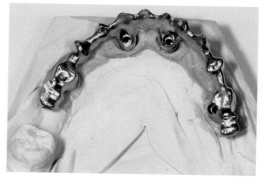

Fig 3-141 Creation of a CAD/CAM-milled framework for an acrylic veneer.

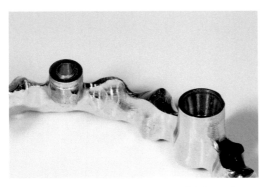

Fig 3-142 Check of the fit on the prefabricated abutments.

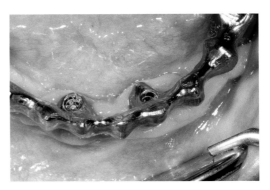

Fig 3-143 Try-in of the framework on the incorporated abutments in the patient's mouth.

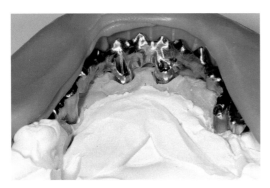

Fig 3-144 Preparation for acrylic veneering with matrix.

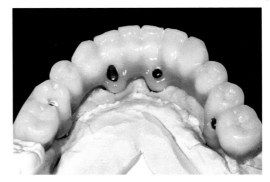

Fig 3-145 Finishing the acrylic-veneered CAD/CAM framework.

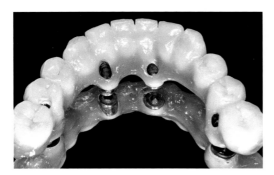

Fig 3-146 Acrylic veneer with incorporated veneers and gingiva-colored acrylic on the basal portion.

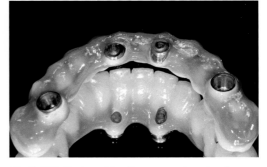

Fig 3-147 Hygiene-friendly concave basal surface.

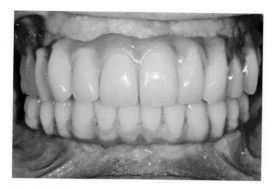

Fig 3-148 Inserted, fixed restorations in the maxilla and mandible created using the SKY fast & fixed method.

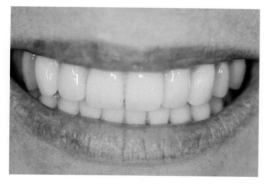

Fig 3-149 Harmonious anterior profile after insertion of the overall restoration.

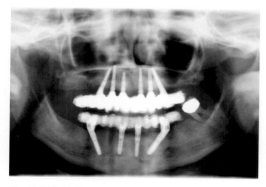

Fig 3-150 Follow-up radiograph of the inserted restoration in the maxilla and mandible.

The universal connector element used with the Landsberger bridge is a prefabricated abutment system with an integrated horizontal screw connection and a titanium coping with a function comparable to that of electroplated copings. Industrially prefabricated parts facilitate and accelerate work and ensure high precision. The predefined adhesive gap of 0.15 mm allows even large bridges to be incorporated with passive fit.

An advantage of this design is that the basal surfaces of the bridge are made of zirconium dioxide and veneer ceramic – two materials with very low plaque affinity[183]. In anterior teeth, customized veneers are essential for esthetic purposes. In the posterior region, the veneers of the visio.lign system, featuring the abrasion behavior of natural teeth, are an optimal system component[61].

In cases of long-segment implant structures in the mandible, the torsion applied to the mandibular superstructure must be considered. However, if the distal implants are inserted at an angle of 35 degrees to the tooth axis, the implant bed lies in the torsion-free area, so that the bridge can be screwed in place without risk.

The following steps are taken before the fabrication of a definitive Landsberger bridge:
1. closed impression-taking accompanied by a radiograph
2. splinting of the impression copings using a customized open tray, setup of the anterior teeth and radiographic check
3. setup and check of jaw relation
4. try-in of setup with an acrylic bridge body that reproduces the definitive size, shape and color
5. fabrication of a metal control key with splinted impression posts
6. patient evaluation of the setup.

If the setup corresponds to the patient's wishes, fabrication of the bridge can begin. To condition the zirconium dioxide framework, a glaze containing aluminium oxide particles is applied to the posterior region and glazed on the framework at approximately 1,000 °C. The resulting surface allows optimal bonding of the veneer that is later applied to the posterior region. The ceramic layering is first performed in the anterior region in the usual manner. Once the ceramic veneers are complete, the posterior region is created with composite and veneers; a silicone key is used in this case as well. After all the excess material has been removed, the facets can be fixed by light curing. When a non-transparent silicone key is used, it is recommended to perforate the key and wait for six minutes after light curing to allow deep polymerization. After the key is removed, all sides are thoroughly exposed to light again for further curing. All of the concave sites are now filled with light-curing incisal, dentin or pink composite and light cured. The surfaces are then polished to a high gloss. This procedure results in an optimal esthetic outcome.

With the secondary crown technique, intraoral adhesion is generally preferred. A precise model for extraoral adhesion can be produced, however, by creating keys of the impression abutments on a metal frame as described. Adhering the restoration on this special model is easier and saves time for the dentist and patient and allows bonding to take place under laboratory conditions. The presented method ensures precise fit of the restoration and offers effective control of the esthetic results.

Figures 3-151 to 3-159 show a clinical example of the fabrication of a Landsberger bridge.

3.7.5 Customized milled bar with removable bridge

Most patients desire fixed restorations. When there is a significant loss of substance, however, a bridge may not offer the necessary support for the lip and cheek area. In these cases, a customized bar with latches or attachments can be a good alternative for use with the presented system.

SKY fast & fixed abutments are designed for primary splinted structures and are hence suitable for bar constructions; for instance, in combination with the SKY bar system.

The procedure is otherwise the same as that described for the Landsberger bridge.

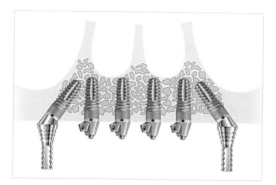

Fig 3-151 In restorations with a Landsberger bridge, the terminal abutments are not changed for the definitive superstructure.

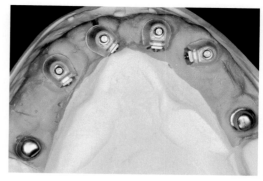

Fig 3-152 Horizontally screwed abutments (universal connector element copings) are placed on the mesial implants, which are bonded to the zirconium dioxide framework with stress-free (passive) fit.

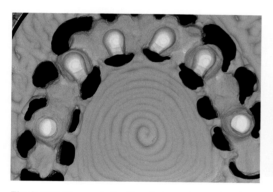

Fig 3-153 The seats for the abutments can be clearly seen in the milled-out underside of the framework.

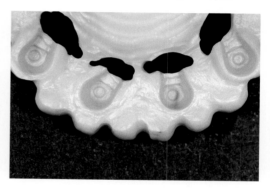

Fig 3-154 The colored and sintered zirconium dioxide framework with the milled-out seats for the laterally screwed abutments.

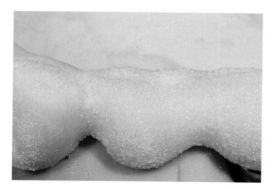

Fig 3-155 Ceramic veneer is applied to the framework in the anterior region, and veneers are bonded to the framework in the posterior region.

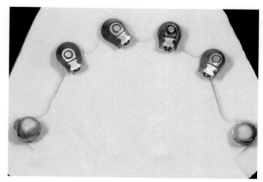

Fig 3-156 A special adhesive model is created for the stress-free bonding of the abutment to the framework.

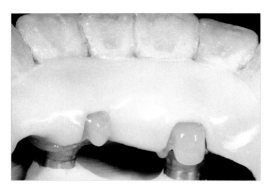

Fig 3-157 After conditioning the zirconium dioxide framework, stress-free bonding of the abutments can be performed on the adhesive model as it would in the mouth.

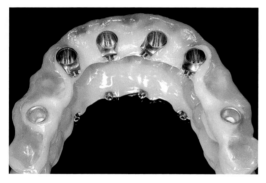

Fig 3-158 The convex-based zirconium dioxide framework with bonded abutments polished to a high gloss.

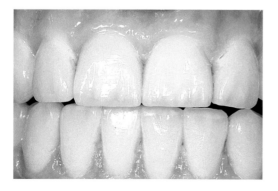

Fig 3-159 During insertion, the abutment screws are tightened to 25 Ncm, and the lateral screws are tightened hand-tight.

3.7.6 Additional restoration options

The restorations described in the above sections are not the only options available with the SKY fast & fixed method. Customized NPM bars milled with the aid of CAD/CAM systems and, under certain circumstances, telescopic crowns are also suitable for restorations with angled posterior implants. When there is a significant loss of substance, it can be difficult to improve the extra-oral esthetics with fixed restorations. However, the patient's wishes may be satisfied using a removable denture on a bar or on telescopic crowns. In addition, such structures can take into account age-related limitations of the patient's manual dexterity. Milled bars, represent a modern alternative to cast bars. Independent or industrially operated milling centers are available for producing such bars as well as milled NPM, titanium or zirconium bridge frameworks for fixed superstructures. In this case, the laboratory is responsible for design. Depending on the employed procedure, the milling center is given a mock-up to be scanned in or is sent the scan data from the laboratory. The proposed framework design is then coordinated with the dental technician, who is responsible for approving it.

Under these conditions, the SKY fast & fixed method can also be used to satisfy unusual patient wishes, such as those of a 70-year-old patient who wanted a fixed restoration in the maxilla and mandible that could be converted into a removable denture at any time without major effort. This patient's wishes were accommodated to her great satisfaction using a provisionally bonded bridge on telescopic crowns over customized abutments (Figs 3-160 to 3-192).

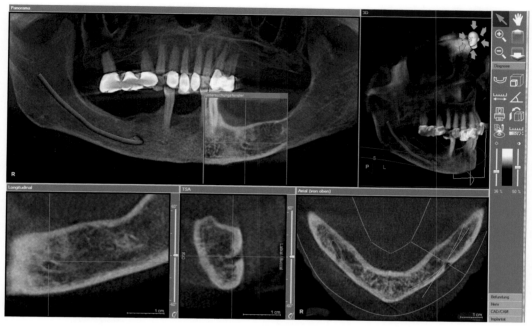

Fig 3-160 DVT images for assessing the retainability of dentition with periodontal damage.

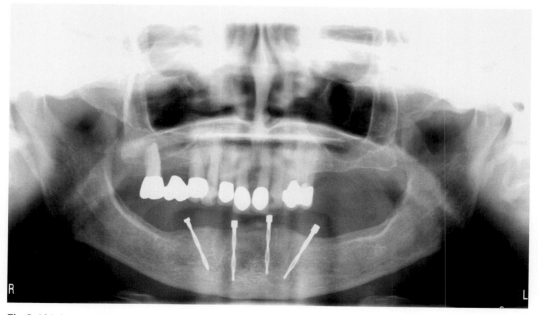

Fig 3-161 Intraoperative radiographic image for measurement purposes, distinctly showing the course of the mental nerve loop.

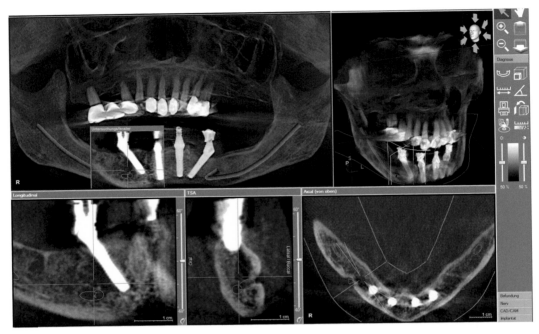

Fig 3-162 Postoperative radiological follow-up of the anatomical structures.

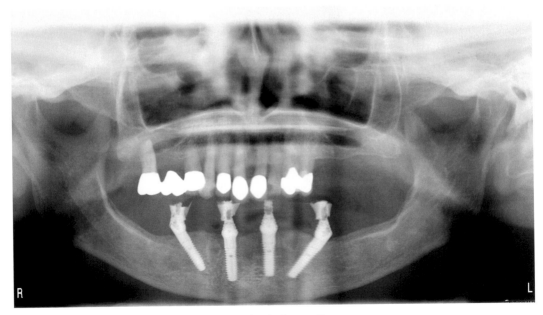

Fig 3-163 Radiological follow-up before implantation in the maxilla.

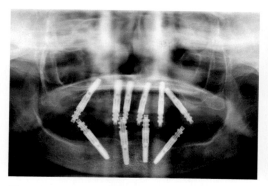

Fig 3-164 Initial situation for a definitive restoration in the maxilla and mandible with a composite-veneered zirconium bridge (illustrating the maxillary restoration).

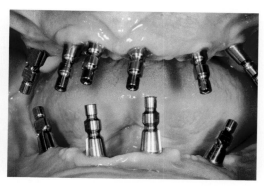

Fig 3-165 Inserted impression abutments for the closed alginate impression.

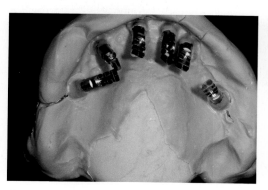

Fig 3-166 Alginate impression for preparing the impression over the primary-splinted impression abutments.

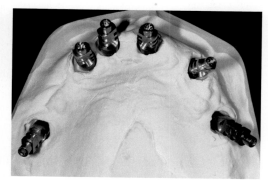

Fig 3-167 The impression abutments for the closed impression were replaced with the impression abutments for the open impression.

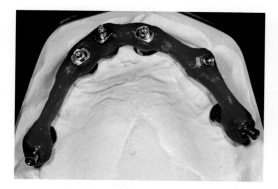

Fig 3-168 The impression abutments for the open impression are splinted.

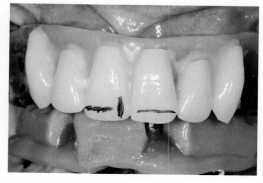

Fig 3-169 After the bite check, the first try-in allows the correction of tooth shape and position in consultation with the patient.

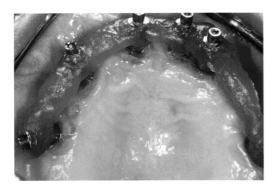

Fig 3-170 The tension-free seating is checked intraorally, and the previously sectioned plastic bar is splinted again in the mouth.

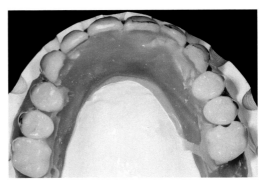

Fig 3-171 After the impression is taken for the master model, the setup can be screwed onto the implants for the esthetic try-in.

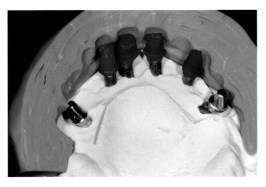

Fig 3-172 The arrangement of the individual abutments is regularly checked with reference to the matrix on the setup.

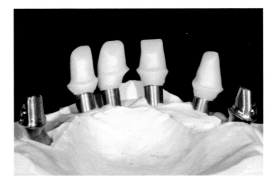

Fig 3-173 The completed abutments are converted into zirconium.

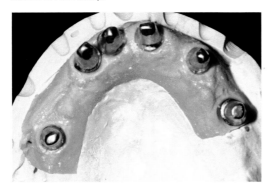

Fig 3-174 After the electroformed copings are placed on the abutments, the setup is cast in resin, and the bridge is ground into the proper shape.

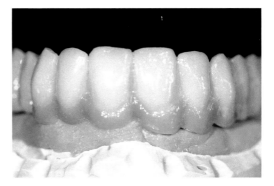

Fig 3-175 The finished bridge undergoes a final esthetic and phonetic try-in.

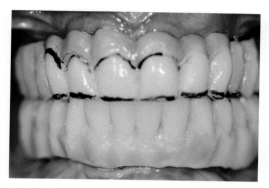

Fig 3-176 Proper occlusion has been achieved, and the desired shortening of the anterior teeth can be achieved visually by modifying the pink portion.

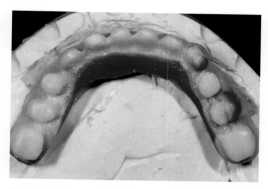

Fig 3-177 The acrylic bridge is duplicated and then reduced be kept as a check model.

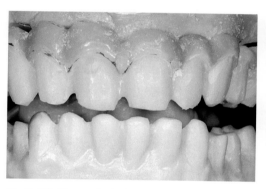

Fig 3-178 The vertical relationship is captured with a silicone stamp.

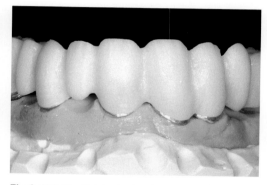

Fig 3-179 The finished setup is converted 1:1 into a zirconium dioxide framework.

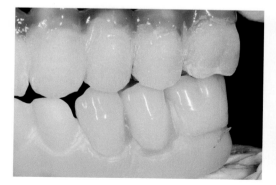

Fig 3-180 In the posterior region, composite teeth are fastened to the ceramic framework, which is basally colored, and composite is layered onto the anterior region.

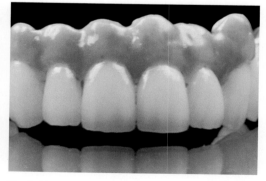

Fig 3-181 The restoration is individualized, reflecting the patient's age.

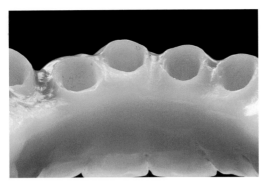

Fig 3-182 The basal surface features the seats for the gold female parts that are bonded stress-free, in this case provisionally.

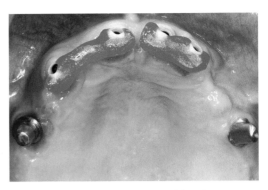

Fig 3-183 For precise alignment of the abutments, the dental technician creates insertion aids.

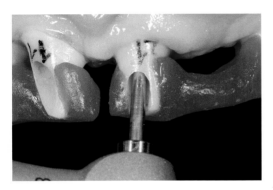

Fig 3-184 The individual zirconium abutments are tightened to 25 Ncm.

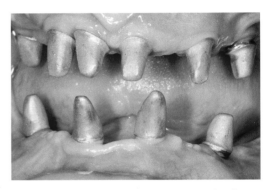

Fig 3-185 Gold female parts mounted on the zirconium male parts for intraoral bonding.

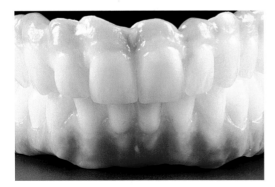

Fig 3-186 A naturally appearing restoration in accordance with the patient's wishes.

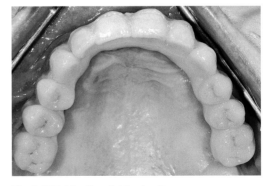

Fig 3-187 Maxillary bridge in situ.

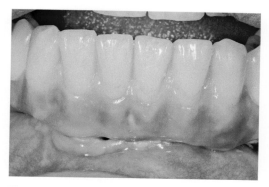

Fig 3-188 The mandibular bridge transitions into the natural soft tissue without any change in color.

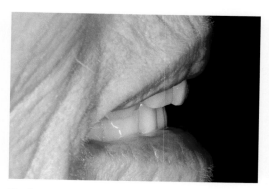

Fig 3-189 A dynamic lip line supported by the restoration...

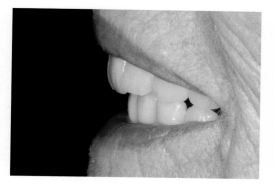

Fig 3-190 ... for an attractive, ageless extraoral appearance.

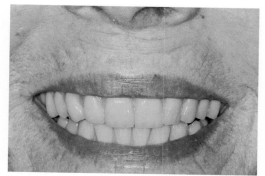

Fig 3-191 The shape and position of the teeth blend harmoniously with the surrounding facial region and give the patient a youthful smile.

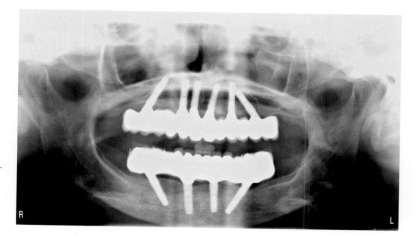

Fig 3-192 A follow-up OPG two years postoperatively in the mandible and 1.5 years postoperatively in the maxilla reveals a stable bone situation.

The presented method is also appropriate when only one side of the jaw is atrophied and requires treatment. Instead of using a clamp-retained denture and exposing the remaining healthy teeth with manageable periodontal problems to the risk of overloading and its consequences, the SKY fast & fixed method can be used to protect the remaining dentition from additional atrophy (Fig 3-193 to 3-207).

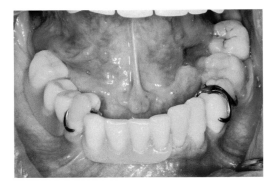

Fig 3-193 Defective dentition with a clasp-retained denture in the fourth quadrant.

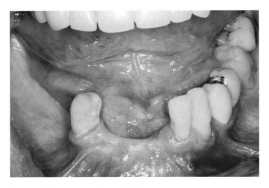

Fig 3-194 Teeth 43 and 32 presented significant looseness so had to be extracted.

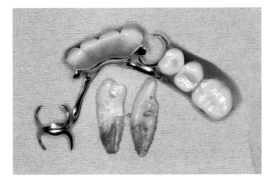

Fig 3-195 Inadequate old prosthesis and extracted teeth.

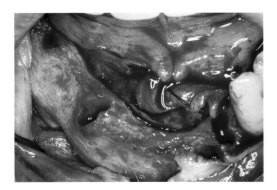

Fig 3-196 Mucoperiosteal flaps created to expose the alveolar ridge and the mental foramen.

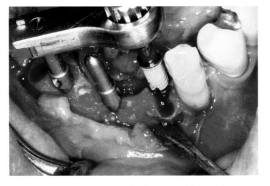

Fig 3-197 The same surgical protocol is used except that only one distal implant is inserted.

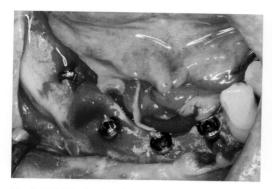

Fig 3-198 The implant in the anterior region is orally offset in the extraction alveolus and possesses primary stability like the other implants.

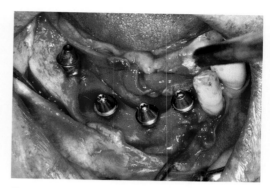

Fig 3-199 The abutments for the temporary restoration are tightened, and the bone defect at position 32 is filled using bone chips obtained from the alveolar ridge.

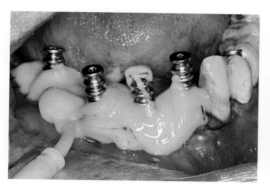

Fig 3-200 Resin is injected around the impression copings in preparation for the impression.

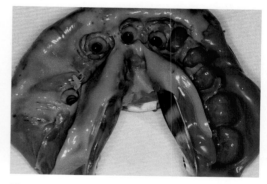

Fig 3-201 Precise impression taking is essential for the restoration to fit well.

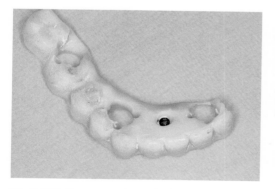

Fig 3-202 The prepared prosthetic body with a previously attached prosthetic coping and spaces for the other prosthetic copings.

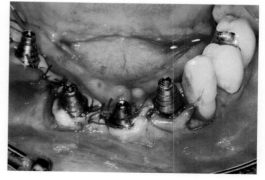

Fig 3-203 The other prosthetic copings are fixed in the mouth with stress-free (passive) fit.

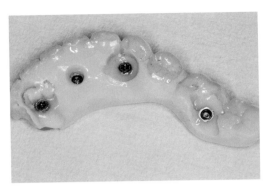

Fig 3-204 After intraoral fixation the prosthetic copings are filled.

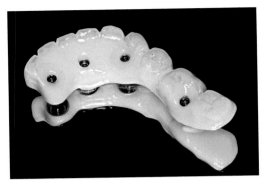

Fig 3-205 The occlusal surface and base of the bridge are finished and polished to a high gloss.

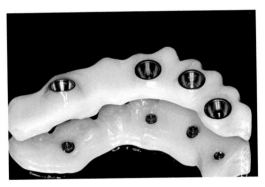

Fig 3-206 The temporary restoration is now ready to be incorporated.

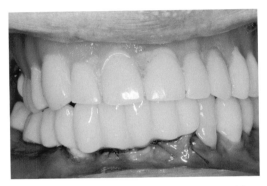

Fig 3-207 Just a few hours after surgery, the bridge can be screwed in place in the patient's mouth.

4 Patient satisfaction

Satisfied patients are the most important assets of any dental practice. Patient satisfaction can be measured directly via objective findings from examination as well as via the patient's immediate response both during treatment and after its completion. Patient surveys are an additional tool for measuring the degree of satisfaction. Patients' assessments of the success of treatment depend on the clinical results and on complications that arose during treatment. Their willingness to incur additional treatment expenses is influenced by their expectations and by the dentist's patient guidance. In an effort to assess the subjective parameters for the SKY fast & fixed method, a patient survey was taken in the context of follow-up examinations at least six months after incorporation of the definitive restoration.

4.1 Postoperative complications

The observed postoperative complications did not noticeably differ from those found in conventional implant treatment. However, it should be noted that this method involves more extensive treatment as a result of the transgingival approach and the immediate restoration. During treatment planning and surgery, it is particularly important to correctly identify the configuration of the mental foramen to avoid damaging the mental nerve[68].

Since the SKY fast & fixed approach targets a patient group with high rates of pre-existing damage resulting from periodontal disease or heavy nicotine consumption, the risk of wound healing problems is increased[136]. These problems primarily involve suture dehiscence, which often heals without further complications when found over local bone or autologous augmentation material[120]. In cases of large ruptures or the use of xenogeneic bone grafting material for augmentation, extensive tissue necrosis can arise, requiring additional therapy. Remobilizing the flap is not a promising option, since the regeneration potential of the already bradytrophic tissue is very limited after another surgical procedure and because of the risk of further necrosis. Wound healing also requires treatment of the local infection. The treatment of peri-implantitis has shown that antimicrobial photodynamic therapy (aPDT)

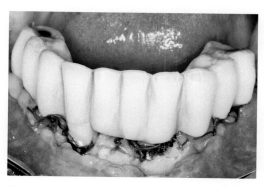

Fig 4-1 Extensive wound dehiscence 10 days postoperatively in a patient with continued heavy nicotine consumption.

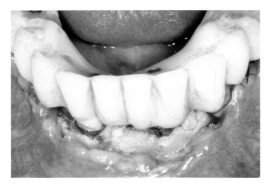

Fig 4-2 Wound cleaning and suture removal with a wide zone of exposed bone.

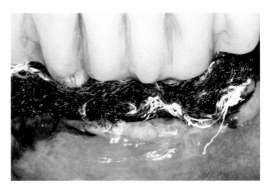

Fig 4-3 Application of the HELBO® photosensitizer with gauze strips for staining the infected areas.

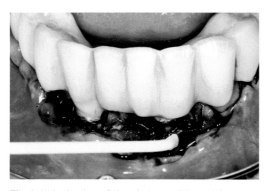

Fig 4-4 Activation of the photosensitizer with a HELBO® TheraLite low-level laser.

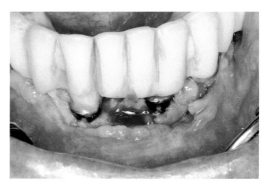

Fig 4-5 Incipient secondary granulation after five days, before additional HELBO® disinfection.

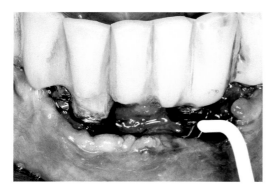

Fig 4-6 Repeat aPDT to decontaminate the exposed bone and support secondary granulation.

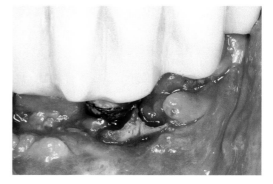

Fig 4-7 Extensive granulation with necrotic bone at implant 32, which is piezosurgically osteotomized.

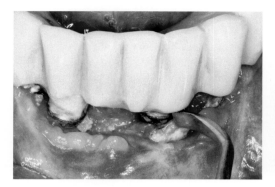

Fig 4-8 Mobile sequestrum before removal.

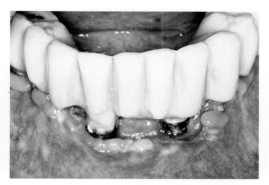

Fig 4-9 Complete granulation three weeks after suture removal and four sessions of aPDT.

can successfully decontaminate the infected area while supporting secondary granulation[117] (Figs 4-1 to 4-9).

In this procedure, the bacterial lipid membranes are stained by applying a photosensitizer to the infected area. After an incubation time of at least 60 seconds, the excess dye solution is rinsed off, and the sensitizer is activated using a low-level laser. This procedure can achieve bacterial decontamination and support wound healing, even at surgical sites[121].

Sequestration can occur as a rather rare, delayed primary complication associated with devitalized bone in the mandible. This complication manifests in the form of small sequestra forming in the alveolar bone surrounding the extracted teeth. In addition to superficial removal, which can be supported by piezosurgery in case of large sequestra, photodynamic therapy is used for wound decontamination in these cases as well[151].

4.2 Late complications

Complications can also arise in the (provisional and definitive) prosthetic restoration phases. If the patient has been partially or fully edentu-

lous for a long time, the stomatognathic system must slowly adapt to the new situation in a functional rehabilitation process. Habitual occlusion, parafunctional habits and temporomandibular problems as well as the functional relation between maxilla and mandible must be considered[136]. Determining an adequate vertical dimension is crucial. Clinical and, if necessary, subsequent instrumental functional analysis reduce the risk of unidentified problems and overloading. The bite may need to be lowered, particularly within the first few weeks after incorporating the provisional, to exclude parafunctional habits and abnormal loads (Fig 4-10).

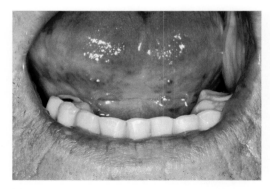

Fig 4-10 Inappropriate vertical dimension with temporomandibular joint discomfort four weeks after surgery.

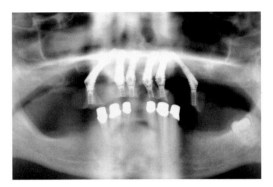

Fig 4-11 Follow-up panoramic radiograph after incorporation of the immediate restoration in the maxilla.

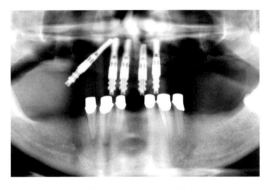

Fig 4-12 Loss of a terminal implant following breakage of the provisional and missed follow-up appointment.

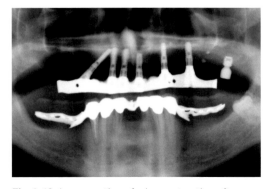

Fig 4-13 Incorporation of a bar restoration after sinus floor augmentation in the left maxilla.

Primarily during the initial restoration phase, and particularly when the size of the acrylic prosthesis is inadequate, abnormal loading can cause instability or even fracture of the provisional and endanger implant osseointegration in the immediate loading phase[49]. Various authors have reported fractures of the definitive superstructures, particularly of the extensions[99,142,193]. Fractures are more common with classic restoration methods than in the SKY fast & fixed approach, where the limited size of the extensions and the specific abutment design almost completely eliminate them. In fact, in recent years, the only fractures have involved inadequately sized precious metal-containing frameworks, and never implants or abutments[2].

In cases of implant loss, another implant can usually be inserted. Depending on the configuration of the defect after examination, however, doing so may require sinus floor augmentation (Figs 4-11 to 4-13).

To eliminate the risk of complications as much as possible, the usual precautions applicable to functional immediate restorations must be observed. Patients must be informed in detail of these decisive factors, in a manner they can understand.

The authors' follow-up study included 314 implants in 66 patients, and the evaluation was performed after the definitive superstructure had been in place for at least one year. The study found that seven implants were lost, resulting in an implant survival rate of 97.3%. Four angled implants and three axial implants were lost, which equates to a survival rate of 98% for the axial implants and 96.5% for the angled implants, with a maximum time in situ of 5.4 years and an average survival time of 2.9 ± 1.17 years (Fig 4-14). The difference is statistically insignificant and confirms that angled implants can be successfully employed[7,102,163]. A total of five patients lost implants, with two patients losing two implants each, one axial and one angled. One patient experienced a relatively late implant loss 2.7 years after implantation. This patient exhibited postoperative problems with wound healing with an extended follow-up treatment period and peri-implantitis therapy, which at that time did not include initial photodynamic therapy. Only one angled implant in the maxilla was lost early, after an initially undiscovered fracture of the provisional. Two mandibular implants were removed, likely as a result of excessive compression of the bone caused by very high insertion torque.

Six patients exhibited inflammation of the peri-implant soft tissue with otherwise symptom-free healing. Peri-implantitis of various degrees of severity arose at 17 implants, of which 11 were axial and 6 angled. All of the complications that arose were treated locally and healed[151].

The collected results illustrate the fundamental importance of regular follow-up visits at an individualized frequency determined by the dentist, especially in the early phase of immediate loading. This gives the patient and the dentist an opportunity to identify infections and defects early on, so that they can be treated without extensive and time-consuming therapy. The treatment approach plays an important role in this regard since reducing the number of implants also decreases the long-term risk of problems arising at individual implant sites. It often takes 5 or 10 years for the long-term clinical results to reveal the effectiveness of the selected method[87].

Despite high success rates and patients' broad acceptance of implants, it is important for everyone, particularly patients, to remain aware that an osseointegrated implant is a foreign body without the self-protecting properties exhibited by natural teeth with periodontium. Repeatedly reminding patients of this fact in a manner that is easily comprehensible will increase the long-term success rate and hence the dentist's recommendation rate.

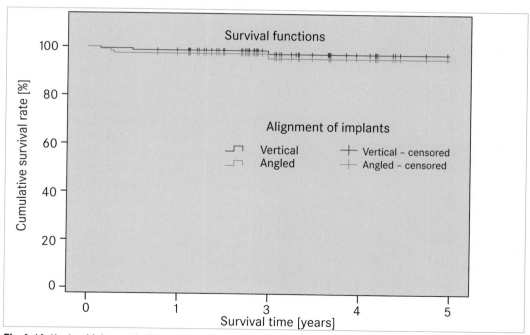

Fig 4-14 Kaplan-Meier survival curves according to implant alignment.

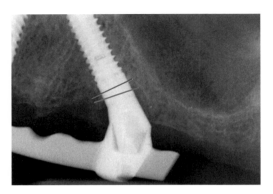

Fig 4-15 Dental film to check the peri-implant bone level revealing a change of 0.8 mm after 2.2 years.

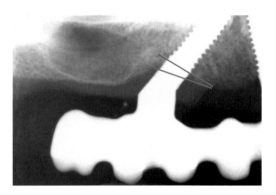

Fig 4-16 Dental film to check the peri-implant bone level revealing a change of 1.9 mm after 2.9 years.

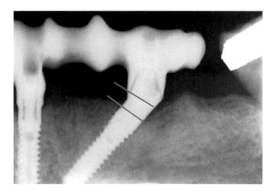

Fig 4-17 Dental film to check the peri-implant bone level revealing a change of 3.1 mm after 1.8 years.

In regard to the changes in the bone level, 15 cases with the implants in place for more than two years were evaluated. The evaluation included 30 angled implants, of which 22 were mandibular and eight maxillary. The average angulation of all the mesial and distal implants was 24.6 degrees. The radiographs were taken after an average loading time of 27.5 months. The point at which the patient received the definitive restoration was used as the baseline. The analysis yielded the following results:

Minor changes of less than 1 mm difference between the bone level and the abutment level were found in 73% of the implants, specifically 18 mandibular and 4 maxillary implants. Five implants, three mandibular and two maxillary, exhibited a moderate change of between 1.5 mm and 3 mm. Extensive changes of greater than 3 mm were found in three implants, one mandibular and two maxillary (Figs 4-15 to 4-17).

These values reflect the clinical experience that peri-implant infections are not found in the absence of significant bone loss.

4.3 Patient satisfaction

A major criterion for patient satisfaction is the degree to which the patient's wishes were satisfied and the predicted results were achieved. When treatment goals are aligned with patient wishes, patient satisfaction is likely to be high, provided that the existing options and risks were thoroughly discussed[53].

Most patients present to the practice with a damaged periodontal system corresponding to a phase 3 bone loss. At that point, augmentation-free restoration of the alveolar ridge can only be achieved prosthetically. The altered implant-to-crown ratio requires a specific procedure with special materials to achieve an attractive appearance and full function. The patient's smile line represents another relevant factor. A high smile line, which is exhibited by approximately 10.5% of patients, presents a great challenge. An average smile line is found in 69.0% of patients and is somewhat less challenging. Only a quarter of patients exhibit an unproblematic, low smile line.

A survey conducted no less than 6 months after incorporation surveyed patients about their prosthetic restoration (Figs 4-18 and 4-19). Such surveys are subject to many limitations, but they still provide useful information regarding patient guidance and organization of the practice[171,172]. Approximately one-quarter of those surveyed reported that the treatment was too long, while the other three-quarters stated that they were "fully satisfied" with its length. Responses to whether esthetic expectations were satisfied were similarly positive – for both the temporary and the definitive restoration. On a scale of 1 for "very good" to 5 for "poor", all

areas were rated "very good" to "good", with two exceptions: Some patients rated the cleanability of the provisional as merely "satisfactory." Beyond patient compliance, this result could be explained by the system-related voluminous design of the provisional, and by being fixed the restorations cannot be removed for cleaning, unlike the old removable restoration for the patient's reduced dentition. This interpretation of the results is supported by the fact that patients do not consider cleanability an issue with the definitive superstructures. The results for "masticatory function" differed somewhat, with lower ratings achieved by the definitive restoration than by the provisional. This result is difficult to interpret. It is likely to be related to patients becoming used to the new restoration. When compared to a previous, inadequate restoration, the difference in masticatory function is quite noticeable. Over time, however the patient be-

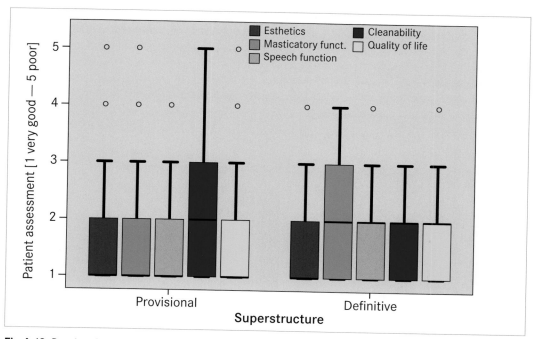

Fig 4-18 Results of the patient survey by the five surveyed criteria.

comes accustomed to the restored masticatory function as achieved by the immediate provisional restoration. The patient then experiences little or no improvement of masticatory function when switching from the perfectly adjusted occlusion of the provisional to the definitive restoration, a fact that is likely to be at the root of this rating (Figs 4-18 and 4-19).

The other criteria, such as esthetics, speech function and quality of life, were all rated "good" or "very good" for both the temporary and definitive restorations. Patient acceptance of the treatment and of the method is impressively illustrated by the responses regarding whether they would choose the treatment again: approximately 95% responded with "yes". This consistently highly positive assessment is also reflected in a question essential to the success of any dental practice: more than 97% would recommend the treatment to friends and acquaintances.

Responses to the question on esthetics in a different study somewhat contradict the above results[53]. Some of the respondents rated the definitive restoration as "average", whereas the provisional was rated "good". This may result from unrealized expectations regarding the appearance of the restoration if its limitations (such as brushing channels, some slightly visible abutments, long crowns, unnatural-looking

gingiva or splinting instead of separate teeth) were not sufficiently communicated before the treatment in a manner understandable to the patient. In addition, patients probably expect less of a provisional than of a definitive restoration. This point needs to be examined in more detail in subsequent surveys.

In view of these results, we conclude that the overall high level of patient satisfaction results from the advantages of the procedure for the patient[3,75]:

- fixed, palate-free restoration, even in the provisional
- no pressure points caused by the provisional
- no second surgery required
- fixed and transparent cost.

The individual comments in the survey (n > 20) additionally indicate a high level of patient satisfaction. In particular, these include positive assessments of:

- the professional and structured treatment process
- the thorough postoperative care
- the fixed temporary restoration.

The majority of patients cited two factors as having decisively influenced their choice of implant procedure:

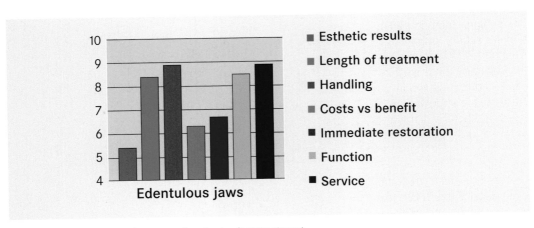

Fig 4-19 Patient expectations regarding the implant treatment.

- less extensive surgery
- reduced overall treatment time.

The positive comments about the professional treatment process also allow the inference that treatment results and hence patient satisfaction are a function of the experience of the dentist-dental technician team and of the effectiveness of their collaboration.

The majority of patients gave a positive rating for the natural and fabricated peri-implant gingiva thanks to the symmetrical pink and white esthetics. The patients' acceptance varied with the selected hue and the successful fabrication of a natural-looking design. In conclusion, the rating in this area also improves with the experience of the dental technician in designing the gingiva in a manner appropriate for the patient's age.

4.4   Results

As mentioned before, the percentage of the population above the ages of 50 and 60 is steadily increasing. As a result, the potential patient population for implant-supported restorations is also growing[66]. However, this patient clientele has a critical mindset, is conscious of the price-performance relationship and is more demanding. Such no patients longer unconditionally accept every suggested therapy but seek out additional opinions and offers, in part motivated by other participants in the healthcare market. The media are becoming more interested in implantology as their audience is inquiring about this therapy and seeks to become informed before making any decisions.

In patients with periodontal damage, the dentition must be critically evaluated to determine how much treatment of the damaged teeth is justifiable[76]. Patients who have chosen or are considering implant treatment usually have very specific expectations: they desire a

fixed and functional restoration as quickly as possible at a reasonable cost, and with minimal surgery.

The classic recommendation of six implants in the mandible and eight in the maxilla with covered healing frequently involves augmentative procedures that are associated with specific risks and longer treatment times[133,148]. It is difficult for the dentist to satisfy patients' demands with this method. Instead, the dentist risks losing the patient or, at best, the patient choosing a different treatment option. To remain successful in implantology, dental practices therefore need options that are adequately tailored to the various patient demands. This is the only way for dentists offering implants to secure their position in the increasingly competitive market.

The use of angled implants with functional immediate restorations is an attractive concept in many regards: It is a very patient-friendly procedure that has already been proven to be practical and suitable for use in dental practices. The logistics of planning are facilitated by precisely harmonized system components. The additional cost of materials for the immediate restoration is negligible. Hence, decisions can be made quickly and easily during surgery. The actual fabrication of a temporary immediate restoration requires a clearly defined amount of time. Finally, the results of the internal follow-up study conducted at the authors' dental practice revealed that the success rates at an average time in situ are similar to those for more extensive surgical treatment methods involving augmentative procedures, such as sinus floor augmentation[141]. In addition, a variety of prosthetic options are available. After the osseointegration phase is complete, telescopic restorations are an option, depending on patient compliance.

All of these advantages represent strong arguments for making such a treatment approach a standard option, provided that patient compliance is thoroughly assessed during the case selection process and that the decision about a functional immediate restoration is only taken after carefully weighing the risks, including during surgery.

Immediately-loaded implants placed and treated under consideration of the cited precautions are not associated with a significantly higher loss rate. Another practical consideration is that patients are more likely to consent to the extraction of problematic teeth as a result of the anticipated treatment results and thereby spare themselves (and the dental practice) much more invasive treatment and a more severely atrophied jaw at a later time.

Patients benefit from a variety of immediate advantages:

- single-session procedure not requiring a second surgery
- as much surgery as necessary, but as little as possible
- fixed, immediately-loaded superstructures, even in atrophied bone
- full functionality, in most cases on the following day
- lower costs at the same level of comfort, thanks to fewer implants
- lower costs as a result of the elimination of augmentative measures
- lower morbidity and minimized risks during surgery
- a fixed price that is easy to calculate for both the dentist and the patient.

Hence, the dentist possesses a scientifically proven and clinically tested approach that allows access to new patient groups and ensures their loyalty over the years.

5 References

1. Adeyemo WL, Reuther T, Bloch W, Korkmaz Y, Fischer JH, Zoller JE, Kuebler AC. Healing of onlay mandibular bone grafts covered with collagen membrane or bovine bone substitutes: a microscopical and immunohistochemical study in the sheep. Int J Oral Maxillofac Surg 2008; 37: 651–659.

2. Aglietta M, Siciliano VI, Zwahlen M, Bragger U, Pjetursson BE, Lang NP, Salvi GE. A systematic review of the survival and complication rates of implant supported fixed dental prostheses with cantilever extensions after an observation period of at least 5 years. Clin Oral Implants Res 2009; 20: 441–451.

3. Al-Omiri M, Hantash RA, Al-Wahadni A. Satisfaction with dental implants: a literature review. Implant Dent 2005; 14: 399–406.

4. Albrektsson T. On long-term maintenance of the osseointegrated response. Aust Prosthodont J 1993; 7 Suppl: 15–24.

5. Albrektsson T, Jansson T, Lekholm U. Osseointegrated dental implants. Dent Clin North Am 1986; 30: 151–174.

6. Anitua E, Carda C, Andia I. A novel drilling procedure and subsequent bone autograft preparation: a technical note. Int J Oral Maxillofac Implants 2007; 22: 138–145.

7. Aparicio C, Ouazzani W, Aparicio A, Fortes V, Muela R, Pascual A, Codesal M, Barluenga N, Franch M. Immediate/early loading of zygomatic implants: clinical experiences after 2 to 5 years of follow-up. Clin Implant Dent Relat Res 2010; 12 Suppl 1: e77–82.

8. Aparicio C, Perales P, Rangert B. Tilted implants as an alternative to maxillary sinus grafting: a clinical, radiologic, and periotest study. Clin Implant Dent Relat Res 2001; 3: 39–49.

9. Assuncao WG, Barao VA, Delben JA, Gomes EA, Tabata LF. A comparison of patient satisfaction between treatment with conventional complete dentures and overdentures in the elderly: a literature review. Gerodontology 2010; 27: 154–162.

10. Bakaeen L, Quinlan P, Schoolfield J, Lang NP, Cochran DL. The biologic width around titanium implants: histometric analysis of the implantogingival junction around immediately and early loaded implants. Int J Periodontics Restorative Dent 2009; 29: 297–305.

11. Balshi TJ, Ekfeldt A, Stenberg T, Vrielinck L. Three-year evaluation of Branemark implants connected to angulated abutments. Int J Oral Maxillofac Implants 1997; 12: 52–58.

12. Balshi TJ, Wolfinger GJ. Immediate loading of Branemark implants in edentulous mandibles: a preliminary report. Implant Dent 1997; 6: 83–88.

13. Becker W, Goldstein M, Becker BE, Sennerby L. Minimally invasive flapless implant surgery: a prospective multicenter study. Clin Implant Dent Relat Res 2005; 7 Suppl 1: S21-27.

14. Beer A, Gahleitner A, Holm A, Birkfellner W, Homolka P. Adapted preparation technique for screw-type implants: explorative in vitro pilot study in a porcine bone model. Clin Oral Implants Res 2007; 18: 103-107.

15. Benzing UR, Gall H, Weber H. Biomechanical aspects of two different implant-prosthetic concepts for edentulous maxillae. Int J Oral Maxillofac Implants 1995; 10: 188-198.

16. Berger C, Engels HB. Kapitel B Qualitäts-leitlinie "Implantologie" des BDIZ. In BDIZ (ed) Indikation enossaler Implantate in Gutachterhandbuch Implantologie, Edition Breisach: Med. Verl.- und Informations-dienste 2002; 59-74.

17. Berglundh T, Lindhe J. Dimension of the peri-implant mucosa. Biological width revisited. J Clin Periodontol 1996; 23: 971-973.

18. Bidgood WD, Jr. Clinical importance of the DICOM structured reporting standard. Int J Card Imaging 1998; 14: 307-315.

19. Binon P. Implants and components: entering the new millennium. Int J Oral Maxillofac Implants 2000; 15: 76-94.

20. Binon PP. The effect of implant/abutment hexagonal misfit on screw joint stability. Int J Prosthodont 1996; 9: 149-160.

21. Binon PP. Evaluation of three slip fit hexagonal implants. Implant Dent 1996; 5: 235-248.

22. Binon PP. Evaluation of the effectiveness of a technique to prevent screw loosening. J Prosthet Dent 1998; 79: 430-432.

23. Boyne PJ, James RA. Grafting of the maxillary sinus floor with autogenous marrow and bone. J Oral Surg 1980; 38: 613-616.

24. Branemark PI, Adell R, Breine U, Hansson BO, Lindstrom J, Ohlsson A. Intra-osseous anchorage of dental prostheses. I. Experimental studies. Scand J Plast Reconstr Surg 1969; 3: 81-100.

25. Brunski JB. Biomechanical factors affecting the bone-dental implant interface. Clin Mater 1992; 10: 153-201.

26. Brunski JB. Avoid pitfalls of overloading and micromotion of intraosseous implants. Dent Implantol Update 1993; 4: 77-81.

27. Calandriello R, Tomatis M. Simplified treatment of the atrophic posterior maxilla via immediate/early function and tilted implants: a prospective 1-year clinical study. Clin Implant Dent Relat Res 2005; 7 Suppl 1: S1-12.

28. Calandriello R, Tomatis M, Rangert B. Immediate functional loading of Branemark System implants with enhanced initial stability: a prospective 1- to 2-year clinical and radiographic study. Clin Implant Dent Relat Res 2003; 5 Suppl 1: 10-20.

29. Canullo L, Iurlaro G, Iannello G. Double-blind randomized controlled trial study on post-extraction immediately restored implants using the switching platform concept: soft tissue response. Preliminary report. Clin Oral Implants Res 2009; 20: 414-420.

30. Chen ST, Buser D. Clinical and esthetic outcomes of implants placed in postextraction sites. Int J Oral Maxillofac Implants 2009; 24 Suppl: 186-217.

31. Chiapasco M. Early and immediate restoration and loading of implants in completely edentulous patients. Int J Oral Maxillofac Implants 2004; 19 Suppl: 76–91.

32. Cibirka RM, Nelson SK, Lang BR, Rueggeberg FA. Examination of the implant-abutment interface after fatigue testing. J Prosthet Dent 2001; 85: 268–275.

33. Clift SE, Fisher J, Watson CJ. Finite element stress and strain analysis of the bone surrounding a dental implant: effect of variations in bone modulus. Proc Inst Mech Eng [H] 1992; 206: 233–241.

34. Cochran DL, Morton D, Weber HP. Consensus statements and recommended clinical procedures regarding loading protocols for endosseous dental implants. Int J Oral Maxillofac Implants 2004; 19 Suppl: 109–113.

35. Conrad HJ, Pesun IJ, DeLong R, Hodges JS. Accuracy of two impression techniques with angulated implants. J Prosthet Dent 2007; 97: 349–356.

36. Cooper LF, Ellner S, Moriarty J, Felton DA, Paquette D, Molina A, Chaffee N, Asplund P, Smith R, Hostner C. Three-year evaluation of single-tooth implants restored 3 weeks after 1-stage surgery. Int J Oral Maxillofac Implants 2007; 22: 791–800.

37. Cunha-Cruz J, Hujoel PP, Kressin NR. Oral health-related quality of life of periodontal patients. J Periodontal Res 2007; 42: 169–176.

38. d'Hoedt B, Schulte W. A comparative study of results with various endosseous implant systems. Int J Oral Maxillofac Implants 1989; 4: 95–105.

39. Danza M, Quaranta A, Carinci F, Paracchini L, Pompa G, Vozza I. Biomechanical evaluation of dental implants in D1 and D4 bone by Finite Element Analysis. Minerva Stomatol 2010; 59: 305–313.

40. Davies JE. In vitro modeling of the bone/ implant interface. Anat Rec 1996; 245: 426–445.

41. Davies JE. Mechanisms of endosseous integration. Int J Prosthodont 1998; 11: 391–401.

42. Degidi M, Piattelli A. Bone-to-implant contact on human retrieval of grid-blasted and high-temperature echted surface implants. In Edition Bologna: 2004.

43. Degidi M, Piattelli A, Gehrke P, Carinci F. Clinical outcome of 802 immediately loaded 2-stage submerged implants with a new grit-blasted and acid-etched surface: 12-month follow-up. Int J Oral Maxillofac Implants 2006; 21: 763–768.

44. Degidi M, Piattelli A, Gehrke P, Felice P, Carinci F. Five-year outcome of 111 immediate nonfunctional single restorations. J Oral Implantol 2006; 32: 277–285.

45. Degidi M, Piattelli A, Iezzi G, Carinci F. Retrospective study of 200 immediately loaded implants retaining 50 mandibular overdentures. Quintessence Int 2007; 38: 281–288.

46. Degidi M, Scarano A, Iezzi G, Piattelli A. Histologic analysis of an immediately loaded implant retrieved after 2 months. J Oral Implantol 2005; 31: 247–254.

47. Del Fabbro M, Rosano G, Taschieri S. Implant survival rates after maxillary sinus augmentation. Eur J Oral Sci 2008; 116: 497–506.

48. Del Fabbro M, Testori T, Francetti L, Taschieri S, Weinstein R. Systematic review of survival rates for immediately loaded dental implants. Int J Periodontics Restorative Dent 2006; 26: 249–263.

49. den Hartog L, Slater JJ, Vissink A, Meijer HJ, Raghoebar GM. Treatment outcome of immediate, early and conventional single-tooth implants in the aesthetic zone: a systematic review to survival, bone level, soft-tissue, aesthetics and patient satisfaction. J Clin Periodontol 2008; 35: 1073–1086.

50. Di Iorio D, Traini T, Degidi M, Caputi S, Neugebauer J, Piattelli A. Quantitative evaluation of the fibrin clot extension on different implant surfaces: an in vitro study. J Biomed Mater Res B Appl Biomater 2005; 74: 636–642.

51. Ding X, Zhu XH, Liao SH, Tong RF, Fang YM, Zhang L. [Establishment of a three-dimensional finite element model of mandible with dental implants for immediate loading]. Shanghai Kou Qiang Yi Xue 2006; 15: 391–394.

52. Edelhoff D, Florian B, Florian W, Johnen C. HIP zirconia fixed partial dentures – clinical results after 3 years of clinical service. Quintessence Int 2008; 39: 459–471.

53. Emami E, Heydecke G, Rompre PH, de Grandmont P, Feine JS. Impact of implant support for mandibular dentures on satisfaction, oral and general health-related quality of life: a meta-analysis of randomized-controlled trials. Clin Oral Implants Res 2009; 20: 533–544.

54. Esposito M, Grusovin MG, Achille H, Coulthard P, Worthington HV. Interventions for replacing missing teeth: different times for loading dental implants. Cochrane Database Syst Rev 2009; CD003878.

55. Esposito M, Grusovin MG, Kwan S, Worthington HV, Coulthard P. Interventions for replacing missing teeth: bone augmentation techniques for dental implant treatment. Cochrane Database Syst Rev 2008; CD003607.

56. Esposito M, Worthington HV, Coulthard P. Interventions for replacing missing teeth: different times for loading dental implants. Cochrane Database Syst Rev 2003; CD003878.

57. Froberg KK, Lindh C, Ericsson I. Immediate loading of Branemark System Implants: a comparison between TiUnite and turned implants placed in the anterior mandible. Clin Implant Dent Relat Res 2006; 8: 187–197.

58. Froum SJ, Wallace SS, Cho SC, Elian N, Tarnow DP. Histomorphometric comparison of a biphasic bone ceramic to anorganic bovine bone for sinus augmentation: 6- to 8-month postsurgical assessment of vital bone formation. A pilot study. Int J Periodontics Restorative Dent 2008; 28: 273–281.

59. Fueki K, Kimoto K, Ogawa T, Garrett NR. Effect of implant-supported or retained dentures on masticatory performance: a systematic review. J Prosthet Dent 2007; 98: 470–477.

60. Gehrke P, Neugebauer J. Implant surface design: using biotechnology to enhance osseointegration. Interview. Dent Implantol Update 2003; 14: 57–64.

61. Ghazal M, Steiner S, Kern M. Abrasionsfestigkeit von Prothesenzähnen. Quintessenz Zahntech 2008; 34: 1016–1019.

62. Glauser R, Ruhstaller P, Gottlow J, Sennerby L, Portmann M, Hammerle CH. Immediate occlusal loading of Branemark TiUnite implants placed predominantly in soft bone: 1-year results of a prospective clinical study. Clin Implant Dent Relat Res 2003; 5 Suppl 1: 47–56.

63. Glauser R, Ruhstaller P, Windisch S, Zembic A, Lundgren A, Gottlow J, Hammerle CH. Immediate occlusal loading of Branemark System TiUnite implants placed predominantly in soft bone: 4-year results of a prospective clinical study. Clin Implant Dent Relat Res 2005; 7 Suppl 1: S52–59.

64. Glauser R, Schupbach P, Gottlow J, Hammerle CH. Periimplant soft tissue barrier at experimental one-piece mini-implants with different surface topography in humans: A light-microscopic overview and histometric analysis. Clin Implant Dent Relat Res 2005; 7 Suppl 1: S44–51.

65. Goodacre CJ, Kan JY, Rungcharassaeng K. Clinical complications of osseointegrated implants. J Prosthet Dent 1999; 81: 537–552.

66. Grant BT, Kraut RA. Dental implants in geriatric patients: a retrospective study of 47 cases. Implant Dent 2007; 16: 362–368.

67. Greenstein G, Greenstein B, Cavallaro J. Prerequisite for treatment planning implant dentistry: periodontal prognostication of compromised teeth. Compend Contin Educ Dent 2007; 28: 436–446; quiz 447, 470.

68. Greenstein G, Tarnow D. The mental foramen and nerve: clinical and anatomical factors related to dental implant placement: a literature review. J Periodontol 2006; 77: 1933–1943.

69. Haas R, Mensdorff-Pouilly N, Mailath G, Watzek G. Survival of 1,920 IMZ implants followed for up to 100 months. Int J Oral Maxillofac Implants 1996; 11: 581–588.

70. Haessler D, Vizethum F, Zoller JE. Autogene Knochentransplantation mit Hilfe eines Spankollectors - eine Methodenbeschreibung. Implantologie 1995; 4: 315–322.

71. Handelsman M. Surgical guidelines for dental implant placement. Br Dent J 2006; 201: 139–152.

72. Hariharan R, Shankar C, Rajan M, Baig MR, Azhagarasan NS. Evaluation of accuracy of multiple dental implant impressions using various splinting materials. Int J Oral Maxillofac Implants 2010; 25: 38–44.

73. Hatcher DC, Dial C, Mayorga C. Cone beam CT for pre-surgical assessment of implant sites. J Calif Dent Assoc 2003; 31: 825–833.

74. Heitz-Mayfield LJ. Peri-implant diseases: diagnosis and risk indicators. J Clin Periodontol 2008; 35: 292–304.

75. Hobkirk JA, Abdel-Latif HH, Howlett J, Welfare R, Moles DR. Prosthetic treatment time and satisfaction of edentulous patients treated with conventional or implant-supported complete mandibular dentures: a case-control study (part 1). Int J Prosthodont 2008; 21: 489–495.

76. Holm-Pedersen P, Lang NP, Muller F. What are the longevities of teeth and oral implants? Clin Oral Implants Res 2007; 18 Suppl 3: 15–19.

77. Horiuchi M, Ichikawa T, Kanitani HR, Kawamoto N, Matsumoto N. Pilot-hole preparation for proper implant positioning and the enhancement of bone formation. J Oral Implantol 1995; 21: 318–324.

78. Hwang D, Wang HL. Medical contraindications to implant therapy: part I: absolute contraindications. Implant Dent 2006; 15: 353–360.

79. Iezzi G, Degidi M, Scarano A, Perrotti V, Piattelli A. Bone response to submerged, unloaded implants inserted in poor bone sites: a histological and histomorphometrical study of 8 titanium implants retrieved from man. J Oral Implantol 2005; 31: 225–233.

80. Israelson H, Plemons JM, Watkins P, Sory C. Barium-coated surgical stents and computer-assisted tomography in the preoperative assessment of dental implant patients. Int J Periodontics Restorative Dent 1992; 12: 52–61.

81. Jensen OT, Shulman LB, Block MS, Iacono VJ. Report of the Sinus Consensus Conference of 1996. Int J Oral Maxillofac Implants 1998; 13 Suppl: 11–45.

82. Jervoe-Storm PM, Hagner M, Neugebauer J, Ritter L, Zoller JE, Jepsen S, Frentzen M. Comparison of cone-beam computerized tomography and intraoral radiographs for determination of the periodontal ligament in a variable phantom. Oral Surg Oral Med Oral Pathol Oral Radiol Endod 2010; 109: e95–e101.

83. Jivraj S, Chee W. Transitioning patients from teeth to implants. Br Dent J 2006; 201: 699–708.

84. Jivraj S, Chee W. Treatment planning of implants in posterior quadrants. Br Dent J 2006; 201: 13–23.

85. Jivraj SA, Corrado P, Chee WW. An interdisciplinary approach to treatment planning in implant dentistry. J Calif Dent Assoc 2005; 33: 293–300.

86. Judy KW. The impact of implants on dental practice. A review of the 1988 NIH Consensus Development Conference. N Y State Dent J 1989; 55: 24–27.

87. Karoussis IK, Bragger U, Salvi GE, Burgin W, Lang NP. Effect of implant design on survival and success rates of titanium oral implants: a 10-year prospective cohort study of the ITI Dental Implant System. Clin Oral Implants Res 2004; 15: 8–17.

88. Keats AS. The ASA classification of physical status – a recapitulation. Anesthesiology 1978; 49: 233–236.

89. Kistler F, Kistler S, Neugebauer J, Bayer G. Implantation im atrophierten Kiefer ohne Anwendung von augmentativen Verfahren – Literaturanalyse und klinisches Vorgehen. Z Orale Implant 2007; 3: 158–169.

90. Klinge B, Meyle J. Soft-tissue integration of implants. Consensus report of Working Group 2. Clin Oral Implants Res 2006; 17 Suppl 2: 93–96.

91. Krekmanov L, Kahn M, Rangert B, Lindstrom H. Tilting of posterior mandibular and maxillary implants for improved prosthesis support. Int J Oral Maxillofac Implants 2000; 15: 405–414.

92. Krennmair G, Furhauser R, Krainhofner M, Weinlander M, Piehslinger E. Clinical outcome and prosthodontic compensation of tilted interforaminal implants for mandibular overdentures. Int J Oral Maxillofac Implants 2005; 20: 923–929.

93. Kupeyan HK, Shaffner M, Armstrong J. Definitive CAD/CAM-guided prosthesis for immediate loading of bone-grafted maxilla: a case report. Clin Implant Dent Relat Res 2006; 8: 161–167.

94. Ledermann PD. Stegprothetische Versorgung des zahnlosen Unterkiefers mit Hilfe von plasmabeschichteten Titanschraubenimplantaten. Dtsch Zahnarztl Z 1979; 34: 907–911.

95. Ledermann PD. Die Neue Ledermann Schraube [New Ledermann screw]. Quintessenz 1988; 39: 799–815.

96. Lindquist LW, Carlsson GE, Jemt T. A prospective 15-year follow-up study of mandibular fixed prostheses supported by osseointegrated implants. Clinical results and marginal bone loss. Clin Oral Implants Res 1996; 7: 329–336.

97. Ludlow JB, Davies-Ludlow LE, Brooks SL. Dosimetry of two extraoral direct digital imaging devices: NewTom cone beam CT and Orthophos Plus DS panoramic unit. Dentomaxillofac Radiol 2003; 32: 229–234.

98. Ludlow JB, Davies-Ludlow LE, Brooks SL, Howerton WB. Dosimetry of 3 CBCT devices for oral and maxillofacial radiology: CB Mercuray, NewTom 3G and i-CAT. Dentomaxillofac Radiol 2006; 35: 219–226.

99. Lulic M, Bragger U, Lang NP, Zwahlen M, Salvi GE. Ante's (1926) law revisited: a systematic review on survival rates and complications of fixed dental prostheses (FDPs) on severely reduced periodontal tissue support. Clin Oral Implants Res 2007; 18 Suppl 3: 63–72.

100. Luterbacher S, Fourmousis I, Lang NP, Bragger U. Fractured prosthetic abutments in osseointegrated implants: a technical complication to cope with. Clin Oral Implants Res 2000; 11: 163–170.

101. Maló P, de Araujo Nobre M, Lopes A. The use of computer-guided flapless implant surgery and four implants placed in immediate function to support a fixed denture: preliminary results after a mean follow-up period of thirteen months. J Prosthet Dent 2007; 97: S26–34.

102. Maló P, de Araujo Nobre M, Rangert B. Implants placed in immediate function in periodontally compromised sites: a five-year retrospective and one-year prospective study. J Prosthet Dent 2007; 97: S86–95.

103. Maló P, Rangert B, Nobre M. "All-on-Four" immediate-function concept with Branemark System implants for completely edentulous mandibles: a retrospective clinical study. Clin Implant Dent Relat Res 2003; 5 Suppl 1: 2–9.

104. Maló P, Rangert B, Nobre M. All-on-4 immediate-function concept with Branemark System implants for completely edentulous maxillae: a 1-year retrospective clinical study. Clin Implant Dent Relat Res 2005; 7 Suppl 1: S88–94.

105. Martin RE. Retiring some myths about aging and oral health. J Gt Houst Dent Soc 1994; 66: 12–15; quiz 16.

106. Meyle J, Gultig K, Wolburg H, von Recum AF. Fibroblast anchorage to microtextured surfaces. J Biomed Mater Res 1993; 27: 1553–1557.

107. Micheelis W, Schiffner U. Vierte Deutsche Mundgesundheitsstudie (DMS IV) Neue Ergebnisse zu oralen Erkrankungsprävalenzen, Risikogruppen und zum zahnärztlichen Versorgungsgrad in Deutschland 2005. Deutscher Zahnärzte Verlag 2006.

108. Misch CE, Wang HL. Immediate occlusal loading for fixed prostheses in implant dentistry. Dent Today 2003; 22: 50–56.

109. Mischkowski RA, Ritter L, Neugebauer J, Dreiseidler T, Keeve E, Zöller JE. Diagnostic quality of panoramic views obtained by a newly developed digital volume tomography device for maxillofacial imaging. Quintessence Int 2007; 38: 763–772.

110. Mischkowski RA, Pulsfort R, Ritter L, Neugebauer J, Brochhagen HG, Keeve E, Zoller JE. Geometric accuracy of a newly developed cone-beam device for maxillofacial imaging. Oral Surg Oral Med Oral Pathol Oral Radiol Endod 2007; 104: 551–559.

111. Mischkowski RA, Ritter L, Neugebauer J, Dreiseidler T, Keeve E, Zoller JE. Diagnostic quality of panoramic views obtained by a newly developed digital volume tomography device for maxillofacial imaging. Quintessence Int 2007; 38: 763–772.

112. Mischkowski RA, Zinser MJ, Neugebauer J, Kubler AC, Zoller JE. Comparison of static and dynamic computer-assisted guidance methods in implantology. Int J Comput Dent 2006; 9: 23–35.

113. Mozzo P, Procacci C, Tacconi A, Martini PT, Andreis IA. A new volumetric CT machine for dental imaging based on the cone-beam technique: preliminary results. Eur Radiol 1998; 8: 1558–1564.

114. Muller W, Lowicke G, Naumann H. [Reconstruction of the alveolar process using molded and compressed spongiosa. A clinical and experimental study]. Zahn Mund Kieferheilkd Zentralbl 1985; 73: 464–470.

115. Mupparapu M, Singer SR. Implant imaging for the dentist. J Can Dent Assoc 2004; 70: 32.

116. Needleman I, McGrath C, Floyd P, Biddle A. Impact of oral health on the life quality of periodontal patients. J Clin Periodontol 2004; 31: 454–457.

117. Neugebauer J. Using photodynamic therapy to treat peri-implantitis. Interview. Dent Implantol Update 2005; 16: 9–16.

118. Neugebauer J, Ritter L, Karapetian VE, Scholz KH, JE. Z. Indikationsbezogene Planung und Gestaltung von Bohrschablonen. Z Oral Implant 2005; 1: 74–81.

119. Neugebauer J, Cantzler P, Piattelli A. 15 Jahre klinische Erfahrung mit gestrahlt-geätzten Oberflächen, die Weiterentwicklung zur CELLplus-Oberflächenstruktur. ZWR 2003; 112: 429–434.

120. Neugebauer J, Iezzi G, Perrotti V, Fischer JH, Khoury F, Piattelli A, Zoeller JE. Experimental immediate loading of dental implants in conjunction with grafting procedures. J Biomed Mater Res B Appl Biomater 2009; 91: 604–612.

121. Neugebauer J, Jozsa M, Kubler A. [Antimicrobial photodynamic therapy for prevention of alveolar ostitis and post-extraction pain]. Mund Kiefer Gesichtschir 2004; 8: 350–355.

122. Neugebauer J, Khoury F, Zöller JE. Influence of the implant surface on the success rate for implants in grafted bone. In Khoury F, Antoun H, Missika P (eds): Bone Augmentation in Oral Implantology. London: Quintessence Publishing Co. Ltd 2007; 67–74.

123. Neugebauer J, Ritter L, Mischkowski R, Zoller JE. Three-dimensional diagnostics, planning and implementation in implantology. Int J Comput Dent 2006; 9: 307–319.

124. Neugebauer J, Ritter L, Mischkowski RA, Dreiseidler T, Scherer P, Ketterle M, Rothamel D, Zoller JE. Evaluation of maxillary sinus anatomy by cone-beam CT prior to sinus floor elevation. Int J Oral Maxillofac Implants 2010; 25: 258–265.

125. Neugebauer J, Scheer M, Mischkowski RA, An SH, Karapetian VE, Toutenburg H, Zoeller JE. Comparison of torque measurements and clinical handling of various surgical motors. Int J Oral Maxillofac Implants 2009; 24: 469–476.

126. Neugebauer J, Shirani R, Mischkowski RA, Ritter L, Scheer M, Keeve E, Zoller JE. Comparison of cone-beam volumetric imaging and combined plain radiographs for localization of the mandibular canal before removal of impacted lower third molars. Oral Surg Oral Med Oral Pathol Oral Radiol Endod 2008; 105: 633–642; discussion 643.

127. Neugebauer J, Stachulla G, Ritter L, Dreiseidler T, Mischkowski RA, Keeve E, Zoller JE. Computer-aided manufacturing technologies for guided implant placement. Expert Rev Med Devices 2010; 7: 113–129.

128. Neugebauer J, Traini T, Thams U, Piattelli A, Zoller JE. Peri-implant bone organization under immediate loading state. Circularly polarized light analyses: a minipig study. J Periodontol 2006; 77: 152–160.

129. Neugebauer J, Weinlander M, Lekovic V, von Berg KH, Zoeller JE. Mechanical stability of immediately loaded implants with various surfaces and designs: a pilot study in dogs. Int J Oral Maxillofac Implants 2009; 24: 1083–1092.

130. Neves FD, Mendonca G, Fernandes Neto AJ. Analysis of influence of lip line and lip support in esthetics and selection of maxillary implant-supported prosthesis design. J Prosthet Dent 2004; 91: 286–288.

131. Nicholson L. Transfer index of multiple angulated abutments in the restoration of an edentulous maxilla. J Prosthet Dent 1997; 78: 605–608.

132. Nkenke E, Radespiel-Troger M, Wiltfang J, Schultze-Mosgau S, Winkler G, Neukam FW. Morbidity of harvesting of retromolar bone grafts: a prospective study. Clin Oral Implants Res 2002; 13: 514–521.

133. Nkenke E, Stelzle F. Clinical outcomes of sinus floor augmentation for implant placement using autogenous bone or bone substitutes: a systematic review. Clin Oral Implants Res 2009; 20 Suppl 4: 124–133.

134. Ormianer Z, Garg AK, Palti A. Immediate loading of implant overdentures using modified loading protocol. Implant Dent 2006; 15: 35–40.

135. Papaspyridakos P, Lal K. Complete arch implant rehabilitation using subtractive rapid prototyping and porcelain fused to zirconia prosthesis: a clinical report. J Prosthet Dent 2008; 100: 165–172.

136. Paquette DW, Brodala N, Williams RC. Risk factors for endosseous dental implant failure. Dent Clin North Am 2006; 50: 361–374, vi.

137. Patil MS, Patil SB. Geriatric patient - psychological and emotional considerations during dental treatment. Gerodontology 2009; 26: 72–77.

138. Perez del Palomar A, Arruga A, Cegonino J, Doblare M. A finite element comparison between the mechanical behaviour of rigid and resilient oral implants with respect to immediate loading. Comput Methods Biomech Biomed Engin 2005; 8: 45–57.

139. Piattelli A, Scarano A, Paolantonio M. Clinical and histologic features of a nonaxial load on the osseointegration of a posterior mandibular implant: report of a case. Int J Oral Maxillofac Implants 1998; 13: 273–275.

140. Piattelli A, Scarano A, Piattelli M. Histologic observations on 230 retrieved dental implants: 8 years' experience (1989-1996). J Periodontol 1998; 69: 178–184.

141. Pjetursson BE, Tan WC, Zwahlen M, Lang NP. A systematic review of the success of sinus floor elevation and survival of implants inserted in combination with sinus floor elevation. J Clin Periodontol 2008; 35: 2 16–240.

142. Purcell BA, McGlumphy EA, Holloway JA, Beck FM. Prosthetic complications in mandibular metal-resin implant-fixed complete dental prostheses: a 5- to 9-year analysis. Int J Oral Maxillofac Implants 2008; 23: 847–857.

143. Rangert B, Sennerby L, Meredith N, Brunski J. Design, maintenance and biomechanical considerations in implant placement. Dent Update 1997; 24: 416–420.

144. Richter U. Der Mentalisloop – Inzidenz und Dimension der mesialen Schleife des Nervus lveolaris inferior auf der Basis computertomografischer Daten. Z Oral Implant 2005; 1: 2–7.

145. Romanos GE. Surgical and prosthetic concepts for predictable immediate loading of oral implants. J Calif Dent Assoc 2004; 32: 991–1001.

146. Rosen A, Gynther G. Implant treatment without bone grafting in edentulous severely resorbed maxillas: a long-term follow-up study. J Oral Maxillofac Surg 2007; 65: 1010–1016.

147. Rosenlicht JL. SwissPlus Implant System, Part 1: Surgical aspects and intersystem comparisons. Implant Dent 2002; 11: 144–153.

148. Sbordone L, Toti P, Menchini-Fabris G, Sbordone C, Guidetti F. Implant survival in maxillary and mandibular osseous onlay grafts and native bone: a 3-year clinical and computerized tomographic follow-up. Int J Oral Maxillofac Implants 2009; 24: 695–703.

149. Scarano A, Iezzi G, Petrone G, Marinho VC, Corigliano M, Piattelli A. Immediate postextraction implants: a histologic and histometric analysis in monkeys. J Oral Implantol 2000; 26: 163–169.

150. Scarfe WC, Farman AG, Sukovic P. Clinical applications of cone-beam computed tomography in dental practice. J Can Dent Assoc 2006; 72: 75–80.

151. Scherer P, Neugebauer J, Karapetian VE, Vizethum F, Zöller JE. Initial therapy of peri-implantitis by anti-microbial photodynamic therapy. In: 20th congress, Association of Dental Implantology, Birmingham, UK: May 3–5, 2007.

152. Schlieper J, Brinkmann B, Metz HJ. [CT-computer-template-assisted planning of implant and magnet position in epi-prosthetic management of facial defects]. Mund Kiefer Gesichtschir 2001; 5: 22–27.

153. Schou S, Holmstrup P, Worthington HV, Esposito M. Outcome of implant therapy in patients with previous tooth loss due to periodontitis. Clin Oral Implants Res 2006; 17 Suppl 2: 104–123.

154. Schulte W, Heimke G. [The Tubinger immediate implant]. Quintessenz 1976; 27: 17–23.

155. Schulte W, Kleineikenscheidt H, Schareyka R, Heimke G. [Concept and testing of the Tubingen immediate implant]. Dtsch Zahnarztl Z 1978; 33: 319–325.

156. Schulze R, Haßfeld S, Schulze D, Ahlers MO, Freesmeyer W, Ackermann KL, Frank E, Terheyden H, Hirschfelder U, Wagner W, Kunkel M, Eickholz P, Edelhoff D, Geurtsen W, Reichert TE. S1-Leitlinie ZMK-Heilkunde Digitale Volumentomografie. AWMF-Reg.-Nr. 083/005 2009.

157. Schupbach P, Glauser R. The defense architecture of the human periimplant mucosa: a histological study. J Prosthet Dent 2007; 97: S15–25.

158. Schupbach P, Glauser R, Rocci A, Martignoni M, Sennerby L, Lundgren A, Gottlow J. The human bone-oxidized titanium implant interface: a light microscopic, scanning electron microscopic, back-scatter scanning electron microscopic, and energy-dispersive x-ray study of clinically retrieved dental implants. Clin Implant Dent Relat Res 2005; 7 Suppl 1: S36–43.

159. Schwartz-Arad D, Gulayev N, Chaushu G. Immediate versus non-immediate implantation for full-arch fixed reconstruction following extraction of all residual teeth: a retrospective comparative study. J Periodontol 2000; 71: 923–928.

160. Scully C, Hobkirk J, Dios PD. Dental endosseous implants in the medically compromised patient. J Oral Rehabil 2007; 34: 590–599.

161. Sennerby L, Gottlow J. Clinical outcomes of immediate/early loading of dental implants. A literature review of recent controlled prospective clinical studies. Aust Dent J 2008; 53 Suppl 1: S82–88.

162. Serra MP, Llorca CS, Donat FJ. Oral implants in patients receiving bisphosphonates: a review and update. Med Oral Patol Oral Cir Bucal 2008; 13: E755–760.

163. Sethi A, Kaus T, Sochor P. The use of angulated abutments in implant dentistry: five-year clinical results of an ongoing prospective study. Int J Oral Maxillofac Implants 2000; 15: 801–810.

164. Silva GC, Mendonca JA, Lopes LR, Landre J, Jr. Stress patterns on implants in prostheses supported by four or six implants: a three-dimensional finite element analysis. Int J Oral Maxillofac Implants 2010; 25: 239–246.

165. Smith DE, Zarb GA. Criteria for success of osseointegrated endosseous implants. J Prosthet Dent 1989; 62: 567–572.

166. Soskolne WA, Cohen S, Sennerby L, Wennerberg A, Shapira L. The effect of titanium surface roughness on the adhesion of monocytes and their secretion of TNF-alpha and PGE2. Clin Oral Implants Res 2002; 13: 86–93.

167. Stanford CM. Dental implants. A role in geriatric dentistry for the general practice? J Am Dent Assoc 2007; 138 Suppl: 34S–40S.

168. Stein W, Hassfeld S, Brief J, Bertovic I, Krempin R, Muhling J. CT-based 3D-planning for dental implantology. Stud Health Technol Inform 1998; 50: 137–143.

169. Steinemann SG, Straumann F. [Ankylotic anchorage of implants]. Schweiz Monatsschr Zahnmed 1984; 94: 682–687.

170. Steveling H, Roos J, Rasmusson L. Maxillary implants loaded at 3 months after insertion: results with Astra Tech implants after up to 5 years. Clin Implant Dent Relat Res 2001; 3: 120–124.

171. Strassburger C, Heydecke G, Kerschbaum T. Influence of prosthetic and implant therapy on satisfaction and quality of life: a systematic literature review. Part 1—Characteristics of the studies. Int J Prosthodont 2004; 17: 83–93.

111

172. Strassburger C, Kerschbaum T, Heydecke G. Influence of implant and conventional prostheses on satisfaction and quality of life: A literature review. Part 2: Qualitative analysis and evaluation of the studies. Int J Prosthodont 2006; 19: 339–348.

173. Strietzel FP, Nowak M. [Changes in the alveolar ridge level in implantation using the osteotomy technic. Retrospective studies]. Mund Kiefer Gesichtschir 1999; 3: 309–313.

174. Strietzel FP, Nowak M, Kuchler I, Friedmann A. Peri-implant alveolar bone loss with respect to bone quality after use of the osteotome technique: results of a retrospective study. Clin Oral Implants Res 2002; 13: 508–513.

175. Sul YT, Johansson C, Albrektsson T. Which surface properties enhance bone response to implants? Comparison of oxidized magnesium, TiUnite, and Osseotite implant surfaces. Int J Prosthodont 2006; 19: 319–328.

176. Szmukler-Moncler S, Piattelli A, Favero GA, Dubruille JH. Considerations preliminary to the application of early and immediate loading protocols in dental implantology. Clin Oral Implants Res 2000; 11: 12–25.

177. Takahashi T, Shimamura I, Sakurai K. Influence of number and inclination angle of implants on stress distribution in mandibular cortical bone with All-on-4 Concept. J Prosthodont Res 2010; 54: 179–184.

178. Tatum H, Jr. Maxillary and sinus implant reconstructions. Dent Clin North Am 1986; 30: 207–229.

179. Testori T, Del Fabbro M, Capelli M, Zuffetti F, Francetti L, Weinstein RL. Immediate occlusal loading and tilted implants for the rehabilitation of the atrophic edentulous maxilla: 1-year interim results of a multicenter prospective study. Clin Oral Implants Res 2008; 19: 227–232.

180. Thomas MV, Beagle JR. Evidence-based decision-making: implants versus natural teeth. Dent Clin North Am 2006; 50: 451–461, viii.

181. Thomason JM. The use of mandibular implant-retained overdentures improve patient satisfaction and quality of life. J Evid Based Dent Pract 2010; 10: 61–63.

182. Tinschert J, Schulze KA, Natt G, Latzke P, Heussen N, Spiekermann H. Clinical behavior of zirconia-based fixed partial dentures made of DC-Zirkon: 3-year results. Int J Prosthodont 2008; 21: 217–222.

183. Trumm W. Ästhetische Prothetik mit Konuskronen. Berlin: Siegfried Klages, 1994.

184. Turkyilmaz I, Company AM, McGlumphy EA. Should edentulous patients be constrained to removable complete dentures? The use of dental implants to improve the quality of life for edentulous patients. Gerodontology 2010; 27: 3–10.

185. Uchida Y, Noguchi N, Goto M, Yamashita Y, Hanihara T, Takamori H, Sato I, Kawai T, Yosue T. Measurement of anterior loop length for the mandibular canal and diameter of the mandibular incisive canal to avoid nerve damage when installing endosseous implants in the interforaminal region: a second attempt introducing cone beam computed tomography. J Oral Maxillofac Surg 2009; 67: 744–750.

186. Van Staden RC, Guan H, Loo YC. Application of the finite element method in dental implant research. Comput Methods Biomech Biomed Engin 2006; 9: 257–270.

187. Van Winkelhoff AJ, Goene RJ, Benschop C, Folmer T. Early colonization of dental implants by putative periodontal pathogens in partially edentulous patients. Clin Oral Implants Res 2000; 11: 511–520.

188. Van Winkelhoff AJ, Winkel EG. Systemic antibiotic therapy in severe periodontitis. Curr Opin Periodontol 1997; 4: 35–40.

189. Watzinger F, Birkfellner W, Wanschitz F, Millesi W, Schopper C, Sinko K, Huber K, Bergmann H, Ewers R. Positioning of dental implants using computer-aided navigation and an optical tracking system: case report and presentation of a new method. J Craniomaxillofac Surg 1999; 27: 77–81.

190. Weibrich G, Buch RS, Wegener J, Wagner W. Five-year prospective follow-up report of the Astra tech standard dental implant in clinical treatment. Int J Oral Maxillofac Implants 2001; 16: 557–562.

191. Weigl P, Hahn L, Lauer HC. Advanced biomaterials used for a new telescopic retainer for removable dentures. J Biomed Mater Res 2000; 53: 320–336.

192. Widmann G, Zangerl A, Keiler M, Stoffner R, Bale R, Puelacher W. Flapless implant surgery in the edentulous jaw based on three fixed intraoral reference points and image-guided surgical templates: accuracy in human cadavers. Clin Oral Implants Res 2010; 21: 835–841.

193. Zitzmann NU, Krastl G, Hecker H, Walter C, Waltimo T, Weiger R. Strategic considerations in treatment planning: deciding when to treat, extract, or replace a questionable tooth. J Prosthet Dent 2010; 104: 80–91.

194. Zitzmann NU, Marinello CP. Treatment plan for restoring the edentulous maxilla with implant-supported restorations: removable overdenture versus fixed partial denture design. J Prosthet Dent 1999; 82: 188–196.

195. Zurdo J, Romao C, Wennstrom JL. Survival and complication rates of implant-supported fixed partial dentures with cantilevers: a systematic review. Clin Oral Implants Res 2009; 20 Suppl 4: 59–66.

Used materials

(All of the materials and methods for which the manufacturer is not indicated are offered by Bredent.)

aPDT	Antimicrobial photodynamic therapy
– Photosensitiser	HELBO®Blue
– Laser	HELBO®TheraLite laser with light guide attachment
Setup	visio.lign veneers
Bridge body	breformance LiquidColdCuring (hot and cold-cure resin)
Fixing cements	Combo.lign, Crea.lign
Disinfectant	Dentaclean (for impressions and prostheses)
Plaster	Thixo-Rock super-hard plaster, class IV
Implants	blueSKY titanium implants
Bone replacement material	ossceram nano, fully synthetic
Bonding agents	Qu-connector and visio.link
Membrane	alveoprotect collagen fleece
Tweezers, diamond-coated	Blue-Clip
Prosthetic resin	Qu-resin, autopolymerizing
Prosthetic teeth	visio.line (neo.ligne full teeth)
SKYplanX	
– Drilling template	3D-resin special resin
– Fixation implants	mini¹SKY FRP
– Scanning template	X-resin CT/DVT, radiopaque resin
– Matrix	brecision Putty soft (hardness: 70 Shore A)
Veneer system	visio.lign veneer system (novo.lign A and P)
Veneer ceramic	GC Initial system for metal, titanium and zirconium frameworks (GC Europe, Belgium)
Matrix	Haptosil D kneading silicone, addition curing (hardness: 90 Shore A)
Gingival mask	
– hard	Exactoform model resin
– soft	Multisil mask